Essential Guide to Blood Coagulation

Edited by

Jovan P. Antovic

Department of Molecular Medicine and Surgery, Coagulation Research, Karolinska Institute;
Clinical Chemistry, Karolinska University Hospital, Stockholm, Sweden

Margareta Blombäck

Department of Molecular Medicine and Surgery, Coagulation Research, Karolinska Institute;
Clinical Chemistry, Karolinska University Hospital, Stockholm, Sweden

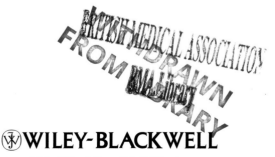

WILEY-BLACKWELL

A John Wiley & Sons, Ltd., Publication

This edition first published 2010, © 2010 by Blackwell Publishing Ltd

Blackwell Publishing was acquired by John Wiley & Sons in February 2007. Blackwell's publishing program has been merged with Wiley's global Scientific, Technical and Medical business to form Wiley-Blackwell.

Registered office: John Wiley & Sons Ltd, The Atrium, Southern Gate, Chichester, West Sussex, PO19 8SQ, UK

Editorial offices: 9600 Garsington Road, Oxford, OX4 2DQ, UK
The Atrium, Southern Gate, Chichester, West Sussex, PO19 8SQ, UK
111 River Street, Hoboken, NJ 07030-5774, USA

For details of our global editorial offices, for customer services and for information about how to apply for permission to reuse the copyright material in this book please see our website at www.wiley.com/wiley-blackwell.

Library of Congress Cataloging-in-Publication Data

Essential guide to blood coagulation/edited by Jovan P. Antovic, Margareta Blombäck.
p. ; cm.
ISBN 978-1-4051-9627-7
1. Blood coagulation disorders.   I. Antovic, Jovan P.   II. Blombäck, Margareta.
[DNLM: 1. Blood Coagulation.   2. Blood Coagulation Disorders.   3. Embolism—physiopathology.
4. Thrombosis—physiopathology. WH 310 E78 2010]
RC647.C55E87 2010
616.1'57—dc22

2009018581

ISBN: 978-1-4051-9627-7

A catalogue record for this book is available from the British Library.

Set in 9/12pt Palatino by Graphicraft Limited, Hong Kong

Printed in Singapore

1   2010

Contents

WARNING: Always check that the prescribed dose is reasonable!

PART 2 Bleeding disorders

PART 3 Thromboembolic disorders

List of contributors

Jovan P. Antovic
Department of Molecular Medicine and Surgery, Coagulation Research, Karolinska Institutet; Clinical Chemistry, Karolinska University Hospital, Solna, Stockholm, Sweden

Margareta Blombäck
Department of Molecular Medicine and Surgery, Coagulation Research, Karolinska Institutet; Clinical Chemistry, Karolinska University Hospital, Solna, Stockholm, Sweden

Katarina Bremme
Department of Women and Child Health, Karolinska Institutet; Obstetrics and Gynecology, Karolinska University Hospital, Solna, Stockholm, Sweden

Anders Carlsson
Department of Medicine, Capio St Göran Hospital, Stockholm, Sweden

Nils Egberg
Department of Molecular Medicine and Surgery, Coagulation Research, Karolinska Institutet; Clinical Chemistry, Karolinska University Hospital, Solna, Stockholm, Sweden

Margareta Holmström
Department of Medicine, Coagulation Unit, Karolinska Institutet; Hematology Centre, Karolinska University Hospital, Solna, Stockholm, Sweden

Hans Johnsson
Department of Emergency Medicine, Karolinska Institutet; Karolinska University Hospital, Solna, Stockholm, Sweden

Rickard E. Malmström
Department of Medicine, Clinical Pharmacology Unit, Karolinska
Institutet; Clinical Pharmacology, Karolinska University Hospital, Solna,
Stockholm, Sweden

Kenneth Pehrsson
Department of Cardiology, Karolinska Institutet; Karolinska University
Hospital, Solna, Stockholm, Sweden

Pia Petrini
Department of Women and Child Health, Karolinska Institutet; Pediatrics
Department, Karolinska University Hospital, Solna, Stockholm, Sweden

Jesper Swedenborg
Department of Molecular Medicine and Surgery, Karolinska Institutet;
Vascular Surgery, Karolinska University Hospital, Solna, Stockholm,
Sweden

Nils Wahlgren
Department of Neurology, Karolinska Institutet; Neurology, Karolinska
University Hospital, Solna, Stockholm, Sweden

Håkan Wallen
Department of Clinical Sciences, Karolinska Institutet; Cardiology,
Danderyd Hospital, Stockholm, Sweden

Preface

The Swedish edition of this book, *Coagulation News*, has existed for over 20 years. It has been re-edited a number of times, more regularly in the past 5 years. This English edition has been rewritten to a greater extent as it includes more medical topics and recent developments in the field.

Essential guide to blood coagulation is a practical guide to laboratory diagnosis and treatment of hemostatic disorders. The book covers both the stable and the acute stages of hereditary and acquired bleeding and thrombotic disorders. A chapter on new anti-coagulants has been added.

Essential guide to blood coagulation is edited in co-operation with physicians now or previously employed at the Karolinska University Hospital (Karolinska), Stockholm, Sweden.

Essential guide to blood coagulation will appeal to interns, hematologists, anesthesiologists, cardiologists, neurologists, pediatricians, laboratory doctors, gynecologists, surgeons, primary care physicians, dentists and students. It can also be used by nurses, hospital chemists, biomedical technicians and midwives.

Jovan P. Antovic & Margareta Blombäck

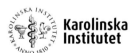 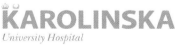

Abbreviations

ADH	antidiuretic hormone
APC	activated protein C
APS	antiphospholipid syndrome
APT	activated partial thromboplastin
ASA	acetylsalicylic acid
AT	antithrombin
AUC	area under the concentration curve
AVK	antivitamin K
BMI	Body Mass Index
BNP	brain natriuretic peptide
CABG	coronary artery bypass graft
CI	confidence interval
CRP	C-reactive protein
CT	computed tomography
DDAVP	1-desamino-8d-arginine vasopressin
DES	drug-eluting stent
DIC	disseminated intravascular coagulation
DVT	deep vein thrombosis
ECT	ecarin clotting time
EDA	epidural anesthesia
EF	ejection fraction
ET	essential thrombocytosis
ETP	endogenous thrombin potential
EVF	extravascular fluid
FDP	fibrin(ogen) degradation products
FPA	fibrinopeptide A
HIPA	heparin-induced platelet aggregation
HIT	heparin-induced thrombocytopenia
HRT	hormone replacement therapy
HUS	hemolytic uremic syndrome
INR	international normalized ratio
ISI	International Sensitivity Index

ITP	idiopathic thrombocytopenic purpura
IUFD	intrauterine fetal death
IUGR	intrauterine growth retardation
LA	lupus anticoagulant
LDA	low-dose aspirin
LDH	lactate dehydrogenase
LE	lupus erythematosus
LMH	low molecular weight heparin
MOF	multiple organ failure
MP	microparticles
MR	magnetic resonance
MRA	magnetic resonance angiography
MRI	magnetic resonance imaging
NSAID	nonsteroidal anti-inflammatory drugs
NSTEMI	non-ST elevation myocardial infarction
OCP	overall coagulation potential
od	once daily
OFP	overall fibrinolytic potential
OHP	overall hemostatic potential
PAI	plasminogen activator inhibitor
PC	prothrombin complex
PCI	protein C inhibitor, percutaneous coronary intervention
PCR	polymerase chain reaction
PE	pulmonary embolism
PKU	phenylketonuria
PLT	platelets
POCT	point-of-care tests
PT	prothrombin time
PTA	percutaneous transluminal angioplasty
RBC	red blood cell
rhAPC	recombinant human activated protein C
rt-PA	recombinant tissue-plasminogen activator
SERM	selective estrogen receptor modulator
SLE	systemic lupus erythematosus
STEMI	ST elevation myocardial infarction
TAFI	thrombin activatable fibrinolysis inhibitor
TAR	thrombocytopenia with absent radius
TAT	thrombin-antithrombin
TDM	therapeutic drug monitoring
TEE	transesophageal echocardiography
TEG	thromboelastography
TFPI	tissue factor pathway inhibitor
TIA	transient ischemic attack

TM	thrombomodulin
TNF	tumor necrosis factor
t-PA	tissue-plasminogen activator
TSH	thyroid-stimulating hormone
TT	thrombin time
TTP	thrombotic thrombocytopenic purpura
UFH	unfractionated heparin
VTE	venous thromboembolism
VWD	von Willebrand's disease
VWF	von Willebrand factor

General hemostasis

PART 1

Schematic presentation of the hemostatic system

CHAPTER 1

Nils Egberg

Department of Molecular Medicine and Surgery, Coagulation Research, Karolinska Institutet; Clinical Chemistry, Karolinska University Hospital, Solna, Stockholm, Sweden

Formation of thrombin via a series of reactions within the coagulation system is central in coagulation activity (Figure 1.1). Coagulation is initiated *in vivo* mainly through exposure of tissue factor, TF, on damaged tissue or endothelium. Activated monocytes can also expose TF, e.g. in sepsis. TF binds and activates FVII. The TF-FVIIa (a = activated) complex initiates coagulation by activating FIX and FX, and they transform prothrombin into thrombin. The process continues, mainly as surface-connected enzymatic reactions, where activated platelets probably offer the phospholipid surface to which coagulation factors (enzymes as well as co-factors) can bind e.g. by means of Ca^2 bridges. Moreover, the coagulation inhibitors (antithrombin, APC) quickly react with nonsurface-connected enzymes and co-factors, which helps to limit the spread of fibrin formation. Thrombin cleaves off fibrinopeptides A and B to form fibrin monomers, which then polymerize and cross-link to form an insoluble fibrin network.

The formation of thrombin is accelerated initially by a positive feedback, whereby the thrombin activates FVIII and FV in order to produce more thrombin. Thrombin also promotes coagulation by activating platelets and endothelium.

The thrombin specificity is modified by its binding to the endotholial receptor thrombomodulin (TM). The TM–thrombin complexes then activate protein C into active protein C (APC), which then decomposes FVIIIa and FVa. So, thrombin both *stimulates and inhibits* its self-formation.

Essential Guide to Blood Coagulation. By Jovan P. Antovic and Margareta Blombäck
© Blackwell Publishing, ISBN: 9781405196277

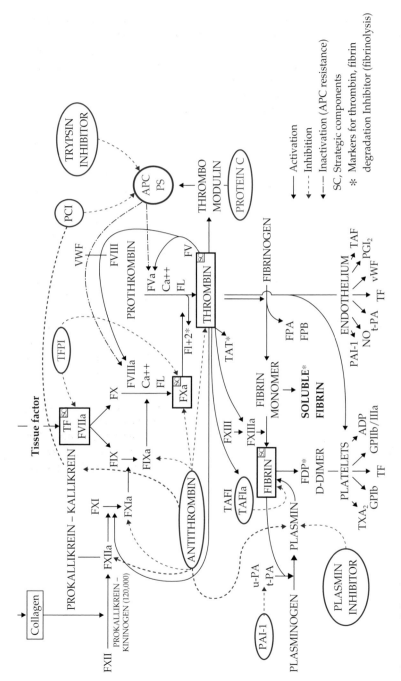

Figure 1.1 Cell and tissue injury.

A model for cell associated blood coagulation has also been proposed where the reaction sequence has been divided into three stages.

- The initiation phase where a small amount of thrombin is generated via the extrinsic pathway to activate platelets and coagulation co-factors V and VIII to their activated forms.
- The priming phase where coagulation factors bind to receptors and phosphatidylserine enriched surfaces on activated platelets.
- The propagation phase where thrombin is formed both via the intrinsic and extrinsic pathways in order to generate large amounts of thrombin that will transform fibrinogen to fibrin.

Antithrombin and APC are the most important coagulation inhibitors. Another is tissue factor pathway inhibitor (TFPI) but its physiologic role is not yet entirely clear. Antithrombin inhibits thrombin by irreversible complex binding, where thrombin-antithrombin (TAT) complex forms. In a similar way, antithrombin also inhibits most of the activated coagulation factors with different affinities. Heparin accelerates the reaction 100–1000 times.

It has recently been discovered that thrombin also has antifibrinolytic effects. It activates thrombin activatable fibrinolysis inhibitor (TAFI) to its active form, thereby inhibiting fibrinolysis.

The activation of fibrinolysis is probably secondary to the activation of coagulation. Tissue plasminogen activator (t-PA) is released from the endothelium and transforms plasminogen into plasmin. The reaction is substantially accelerated by the presence of fibrin, and plasmin formation normally occurs only locally on the fibrin clot. Plasmin breaks down fibrin and fibrinogen into a number of fragments, fibrin(ogen) degradation products, e.g. X, Y, D and E fragments and cross-linked fibrin fragments, fibrin D-dimers. t-PA is inhibited by the release of plasminogen activator inhibitor (PAI-1) from the endothelium. The generated plasmin is bound by the plasmin inhibitor to a plasmin-plasmin inhibitor complex as soon as plasmin is freely present in the blood.

Proposals for sampling instructions

CHAPTER 2

Margareta Blombäck and Nils Egberg

Department of Molecular Medicine and Surgery, Coagulation Research,
Karolinska Institutet; Clinical Chemistry, Karolinska University Hospital,
Solna, Stockholm, Sweden

Points to note prior to sampling

The concentrations of components of the hemostatic system often vary with the patient's condition, e.g. infection, emotional stress, physical exertion (rush to keep an appointment), lipid concentration in plasma, etc.

- *Sitting up/lying down.* Due to changes in hydrostatic pressure, the concentrations of high molecular proteins and blood cells vary according to whether the patient is sitting up or lying down (as much as 15% higher when sitting up). A new balance is reached fairly quickly (15–20 min).
- *Diurnal variations* occur for several factors such as PAI-1 (peaks late at night). Many hemostatic components, such as FVIII, von Willebrand factor (VWF), PAI-1 and fibrinogen, are acute phase reactants (i.e. increased by inflammation, infection, surgery, etc.).
- *Intraindividual variations* occur mainly for FVIII and VWF but also for FVII. Thus, mental stress and physical activity increase the concentrations of FVIII and VWF many times over. Sampling conditions should be standardized as far as possible to minimize sources of error (see below).
- *Smoking and age* affect the levels of several coagulation factors (e.g. VWF and fibrinogen are increased).
- *Estrogen,* high-dose p-pills (and other hormone drugs) also affect coagulation and fibrinolysis (e.g. FVIII, VWF and fibrinogen are increased and antithrombin, protein C and FVII are lowered at high levels of estradiol).

Essential Guide to Blood Coagulation. By Jovan P. Antovic and Margareta Blombäck
© Blackwell Publishing, ISBN: 9781405196277

- *Influence of blood group.* The level of FVIII is about 30% lower in blood group O and the difference for VWF (earlier known as FVIII R:Ag) is somewhat larger. Consequently, levels near the lower reference limit of these factors imply that the patient can be a normal variant or have mild von Willebrand's disease (VWD).

Sampling time and patient preparation

The patient should be calm and relaxed, come to the sampling room without hurrying and sit there for a little while (15–20 min.) before samples are taken.

The patient should have fat-fasted since midnight, or for at least 4 hours. Samples should be taken before 10 am with the patient sitting down. In an investigation for bleeding diathesis, the patient should not have taken ASA or clopidogrel for the last 7–10 days or other antiphlogistic non-steroidal anti-inflammatory drugs (NSAID) for the last 1–3 days. If these drugs have been prescribed, they should not be withdrawn without consulting the physician in charge.

In an investigation of bleeding tendency, fertile women should preferably be sampled during menstrual days 1–4. It is then easier to diagnose a suspected mild VWD. P-pills and other hormone drugs should have been withdrawn, if possible, for at least 1 month. In women who have been pregnant, a deficiency cannot be determined exactly until breastfeeding has ceased and menstruation has become regular. Thus, if these recommendations are not followed, slight defects will seldom be detected.

To monitor the effect of heparin (unfractionated heparin (UFH)/low molecular weight heparin (LMH)) by determining anti-Xa, samples should be drawn 3 hours after an injection in patients receiving "low-dose" prophylactic treatment (1 injection/day) and prior to an injection in "high-dose" treatment (2 injections/day). In treatment that is not prophylactic, samples are usually taken prior to injection.

A coagulation investigation after a thromboembolic complication should be performed, if possible, not less than 3 months after the latest event in order to avoid an acute phase reaction. For example, the amount of antithrombin decreases to about 25% after 4–5 days of IV UFH/LMH treatment. Separate coagulation factor analyses cannot always be performed, since UFH/LMH interferes with the test system. During anti-vitamin K (AVK) treatment, it is not possible to determine the basic levels of the vitamin K-dependent coagulation factors prothrombin, FVII, FIX and FX or the coagulation inhibitors protein C and protein S. If the diagnosis of a hereditary defect is an urgent matter, investigate parents or other relatives with a similar history. The medication is occasionally changed from AVK drugs to UFH/LMH (at least 2 weeks prior to sampling).

If the patient is being treated with AVK drugs or UFH/LMH, you must consider the above. Consult a coagulation expert. *Mutation analyses*, for instance of factor V gene (1691G>A) and prothrombin gene (2021G>A), can of course be performed regardless of whether the patient is on treatment.

Referrals for coagulation analyses

- Give a short case history, the question, results of any earlier analyses and the desired analyses.
- State the sender (full address) and remember to name your hospital and who is to be invoiced.
- Give a combicacode if there is one.
- Always give your telephone/fax number/email if you want a quick reply.
- Always state the date and time of the blood sampling and whether the patient is on AVK drugs, UFH/LMH (even just an occasional flush) or other anticoagulants.
- State if the patient has received a transfusion of blood, plasma or blood products during the past month.

Sampling

Analyses of plasma

- Samples that cannot be analyzed right away must be centrifuged, etc. (see below) and frozen in two portions of 0.6 mL for each analysis in so-called Ellerman tubes at −70°C.
- The outcome of coagulation analyses can be markedly affected by the sampling conditions. The sample should be taken by direct vein puncture, not from heparinized catheters or from an infusion apparatus for administering heparin (UFH/LMH), though see also below. Stasis should be moderate (or nil) and the blood should flow easily.
- *For an investigation of thrombosis and bleeding*, usually four citrate tubes, each containing 5 mL, are taken and the plasma is separated into nine small plastic tubes each containing 0.6 mL. For a single analysis, take one citrate tube and separate the plasma into 3–4 small tubes.
- *For mutation (DNA) analyses:* one EDTA whole-blood plastic tube (5 mL) (if only glass tubes are available, the blood should be transferred to plastic tubes prior to freezing).
- *In sampling from small children,* special 2 mL citrate tubes can be used. Separate the plasma into as many tubes as possible, each containing 0.3 mL.
  For DNA analyses: one EDTA whole-blood plastic tube, about 2 mL whole blood (for handling see above).

Technique

1. The patient should be sitting up. If this is not possible, remember to have the patient in the same position next time so that the results can be compared. Also see above.
2. Take the sample by direct vein puncture, not by an indwelling cannula, with minimal stasis. If an indwelling cannula has to be used, discard the first 5–10 mL of the blood. The first tube cannot be used for coagulation analyses.
3. The blood should flow fast. If not, note the deviations, for instance on the referral.
4. Use 5 mL vacuum tubes intended for coagulation tests (currently siliconized vacuum tubes), containing 0.5 mL of 0.129 or 0.105 mol/L trisodium citrate (9 parts of blood + 1 part of trisodium citrate), pH 7.4. (If blood is taken in open tubes, the proportions of blood/citrate should be the same.) Note that only filled tubes (±10% deviation) are accepted for further handling. For DNA, see above.
5. Reverse the tubes **immediately** 5–10 times.
6. Centrifuge citrate blood samples as soon as possible (preferably within 30 min) at +15°C, alternatively at room temperature for 15 minutes at 2000 x g. Samples for determination of heparin (UFH/LMH) with anti-FXa method (don't forget to state any medication the patient is being treated with) and of lupus anticoagulant must be centrifuged *twice* in order to obtain platelet-free plasma. Note that this plasma can also be used for testing other hemostasis components, such as P-APC resistance, and for research analyses of plasma samples.
7. Centrifuging twice involves pipetting the plasma after the first centrifugation into a new empty tube, which is then centrifuged for 15 min at 2000 x g. The supernatant after the second centrifuging is the test material, i.e. platelet-free plasma.
8. Collect the plasma, *not closer to the cells than 10 mm* (do not disturb the platelets). If there is only one tube of citrate blood, divide the plasma into 0.3–0.6 mL portions in Ellerman-tubes. If there are several tubes of citrate blood, mix the plasma from all the tubes in a separate plastic tube before dividing the plasma into portions, in order to avoid variations in the measured values.
9. Try to get two tubes for freezing for each analysis. Since additional assays often have to be performed, be sure to freeze at least four tubes in order to avoid new sampling. Note this on the referral to the sampling unit.
10. Label the tubes with the date, time, number and name or other identification.
11. Use a rubber band to bundle all the tubes for each patient.
12. Deep freeze the plasma at –70°C within 1 hour after sampling.

For DNA investigation (genetic analysis)

Analyses of mutations of APC resistance – factor V Leiden (1691G>A), prothrombin (2021G>A), FVIII and VWF – are done with the DNA from nucleated cells from EDTA blood. EDTA blood can stand storage in a refrigerator +6°C for about 3 days. It can also be frozen provided the blood (if it comes in a glass tube) is transferred first to a plastic tube. One EDTA tube (5 mL) with whole blood is enough for several mutation assays. Note that the patient should be identified as for blood group testing.

For analysis of fP-homocysteine (EDTA tube)

The tube should be centrifuged within 1 hour (for clinical use). For research analysis the sample should be taken on an *empty stomach*, since food can raise the level 10–15%. Moreover, continuous release from erythrocytes means that the blood cells need to be centrifuged out within 30 minutes. If this is not possible, the sample must be taken on ice. After centrifugation, homocysteine is stable in the plasma at room temperature for several days, so the sample can be sent by ordinary mail. In the frozen state (−20°, −70°) the sample is stable for several months.

Laboratory investigations

CHAPTER 3

Jovan P. Antovic and Nils Egberg

Department of Molecular Medicine and Surgery, Coagulation Research, Karolinska Institutet; Clinical Chemistry, Karolinska University Hospital, Solna, Stockholm, Sweden

Nomenclature

The nomenclature in this book has been adapted from the usage at the Karolinska University Laboratory. It is essentially the nomenclature recommended by the Scientific and Standardization Committee (SSC)/ International Society on Thrombosis and Haemostasis (ISTH), International Union of Pure and Applied Chemistry (IUPAC) and International Federation of Clinical Chemistry and Laboratory Medicine (IFCC).

The most common assays of hemostasis are listed in Box 3.1. The "investigation kit" proposed below may be a suitable starting point. If the analyses do not indicate pathology, additional analyses can be performed. Alternatively, if the patient's symptomatology is indefinite, the investigation can end here.

Box 3.1 Frequently used assays of hemostatic function and hemostatic components

Screening analyses

Pt-bleeding time	P-fibrinogen
CB/B-platelet particle concentration, platelet count	P-fibrin D-dimer
P-APT time	P-antifactor Xa
CB/P-PT(INR)	P-antithrombin
P-factor VIII	Heparin/PF4 antibodies (ID-PaGIA)

Essential Guide to Blood Coagulation. By Jovan P. Antovic and Margareta Blombäck
© Blackwell Publishing, ISBN: 9781405196277

Special analyses

Coagulation factors

P-prothrombin (FII), factor VII, factor X

P-factor V

P-factor VIII

P-factor IX

P-factor XI

P-factor XII

P-factor XIII

P-VWF

Anticoagulants

P-Coag surface-induced antibody – circulating anticoagulants (screening)

P-factor VIII, antibody

P-factor IX, antibody

P-VWF, antibody

P-lupus anticoagulants

Protein C anticoagulant system

P-protein S (free or total)

P-protein C

P-APC resistance

Platelet function

P-platelet aggregation

P-HIPA

P-heparin/PF4 antibodies (HIT) ELISA

Fibrinolysis

P-plasminogen

P-antiplasmin (plasmin inhibitor)

P-t-PA

P-PAI-1

Therapy control

P-antifactor Xa

Markers for coagulation activation

P-TAT complex

P-prothrombin fragm. 1+2

DNA analyses: genetic investigations

Hemophilia, VWD

Factor V genotype (1691G>A)

Prothrombin, genotype (20210G>A)

Notes
- P, measurement made in plasma; S, measurement made in serum; Pt, sample analyzed directly on patient; CB, capillary blood sampling; B, whole blood measurements.
- Strictly speaking, the Roman figure should be preceded by the words "coagulation factor," for example "coagulation factor VIII." If there is no risk of a misunderstanding, however, this can be abbreviated to, for instance, "factor VIII" or "FVIII."
- The prefix "anti-" was often used for inhibitors but nowadays this is done only for components that are antibodies. There are two exceptions: antithrombin (III), which for historical reasons has kept its name, though III has been dropped; and α2-antiplasmin, which has usually kept its former name (the recommendation would be "plasmin inhibitor").

- The old abbreviations of the following components are used in this manual because coagulation specialists have not yet reached a consensus about more appropriate solutions.
  APT time. Should instead be an abbreviation of "coagulation surface-induced time," i.e. the time at activation on a surface.
  P-PT = prothrombin time. Should instead be an abbreviation of "coagulation, tissue factor induced time." It denotes the coagulation time obtained when tissue factor is added to the sample, and measures the sum of the coagulation factors prothrombin (FII) + FX + FVII. The laboratories have currently agreed to use P-PT(INR), as is done in this manual.

Sources:
SSC/ISTH. Nomenclature of quantities and units in thrombosis and haemostasis. *Thromb Haemostas* 1994;**71**:375–394.
Properties and units in the clinical laboratory sciences. V. Properties and units in thrombosis and haemostasis. *Pure Appl Chem* 1997;**69**(5):1043–1079.
An updated version can be found at: www.IUPAC.ORG/publications/pac/1997/pdf/6905x1043.pdf.

In the event of problems in interpreting the analyses or deciding what to do next, contact your own coagulation laboratory or the hospital's coagulation unit in order to discuss.

Reference intervals for laboratory investigations

Consult your laboratory.

Screening analyses

Screening analyses undertaken in hemostatic contexts usually include CB/B-PLT, P-APT time, CB/P-PT(INR), P-fibrinogen and, if applicable, Pt-bleeding time. If disseminated intravascular coagulation (DIC) is suspected, usually P-fibrin D-dimer and P-antithrombin are also measured (P-factor VIII can also be determined). P-heparin/PF4 antibodies (ID-PaGIA) are used for screening and ruling out heparin-induced thrombocytopenia (HIT) diagnosis.

Pt-Bleeding time
Reflects a defect in primary hemostasis, e.g. blood vessel and platelet function. Bleeding time is usually measured with an incision on the lower arm (modified Ivy – ask your laboratory).

Note: Measurement of bleeding time is difficult to standardize and must therefore be performed by skilled personnel. Several investigations show that it cannot be used to predict bleeding during surgery. There is an intraindividual variation in bleeding time. Bleeding time increases with decreasing EVF (hematocrit), e.g. during pregnancy (normally not above the upper reference range). So-called isolated increased bleeding time also occurs (all other tests normal).

Other proposed analyses when bleeding time is increased in spite of normal platelet count

Exclude drug effects (acetylsalicylic acid (ASA), clopidogrel, NSAID). Complete with the following:

- von Willebrand factor antigen/functional assay
- confirm the increased bleeding time
- in severe cases, possibly also platelet function tests, e.g. platelet aggregation test.

Treatment with desmopressin can shorten bleeding time and improve hemostasis, see Chapter 4.

B/CB-PLT (platelet particle concentration = platelet count)

A sufficient number of platelets is a requirement for good primary hemostasis.

Thrombocytopenia is a condition in which platelet count is below 150×10^9/L. It can be hereditary or acquired (see Chapter 4). An increased risk for bleeding is rare at platelet count above 50×10^9/L. The risk of bleeding is often increased at lower levels than that (particularly below 20 and especially below 10×10^9/L). Platelet concentrate is usually needed at considerably lower levels. The risk of bleeding increases as platelet function decreases and/or fibrinolysis increases.

Thrombocytosis is a condition in which platelet count is above 400×10^9/L and may be associated with either thrombosis or bleeding risk.

P-APT (activated partial thromboplastin) time

Reflects a defect in the part of the hemostatic system initiated by surface activation, previously called the "intrinsic coagulation system." Increased APT time is seen in deficiencies of FXII (all levels), FXI, prokallikrein, FIX, FVIII, FX, FV, prothrombin and fibrinogen. In the latter deficiencies, the APT time does not increase unless the deficiencies are severe or moderately severe. The APT time can be normal even at factor concentrations 15–30% of normal (0.15–0.30 IU/mL).

Specific coagulation factor analyses should be performed if a disturbance is suspected clinically even though APT time is normal.

APT time is *not prolonged* in deficiency of FVII or FXIII. APT time is *often prolonged* in the presence of lupus anticoagulant/phospholipid antibodies.

B/CB prothrombin complex

Reflects a defect in the system or systems activated by the tissue factor. This used to be called the "extrinsic coagulation system."

The so-called prothrombin complex consists of prothrombin (FII), FVII, FIX and FX. These coagulation factors are formed in the liver and for their synthesis are dependent on vitamin K. The common methods in Scandinavia and Japan measure the sum of the above-mentioned factor activities, except for factor IX. The prothrombin complex (PC) can be determined in blood (B), capillary blood (kB) and plasma (P).

Prothrombin time (PT) methods vary throughout the world. Most laboratories use simple thromboplastin reagents (Quick "plain reagents"), in which case the test is also dependent on the contents of FV and fibrinogen in the patient's plasma. Adsorbed bovine plasma containing these factors is added to the Owren's reagent ("combined reagents"). The combined reagents are mostly easier to standardize.

PT(INR)

Because all reagents, Quick as well as Owren reagents, contain different thromboplastins, the characteristics of these measuring methods tend to differ. However, the numerical value of a test can be compared with another test with the aid of an international thromboplastin standard, against which every new reagent must be calibrated.

This procedure enables us to express test results as an international normalized ratio (INR). Log INR = ISI × log patient's coagulation time/reference plasma's coagulation time. Alternatively, INR = (patient's coagulation time/reference plasma's coagulation time)^{ISI}.

The International Sensitivity Index (ISI) is an experimentally obtained value for every reagent-instrument combination in use. The ISI value for thromboplastin reagents is recommended to be close to 1.0, which is ideal. INR was adopted by the SSC of the ISTH in 1999. The reference value for PT(INR) is <1.2 (equivalent to over 67% on the earlier percentage scale).

A full list of all comparisons can be found on the Equalis website: www.equalis.se/INR.

PT determinations expressed in INR are internationally accepted only for control of AVK treatment under stable conditions. Experience indicates that results expressed as INR can also be used for estimating liver function or other types of influence on the measurement system.

Spontaneous increase in PT(INR)

Check liver status. Complete with FVII, FX and FII (prothrombin) determinations, and determination of cardiolipin antibodies/lupus anticoagulant. If results disagree, contact a coagulation specialist.

Intravenous injection of vitamin K will normalize P-PT(INR) at deranged adsorptions and in AVK treatment. Note that the full effect occurs after at least 12–16 hours in adults but after just a couple of hours in newborns. Normalization seldom occurs if the liver is damaged.

Note that increased PT(INR) can indicate a corresponding fall in FVII, to which the test is normally most sensitive. On the other hand, deficiency of prothrombin or FX can be more serious than shown by PT(INR) (e.g. FX 0.20 E/mL = PT(INR) 1.3).

P-fibrinogen

Decreased concentration of fibrinogen (below 1 g/L) can cause bleeding. It may occur due to increased consumption/degradation in serious DIC or due to decreased synthesis in evident damage to the liver.

Hereditary fibrinogen deficiency or fibrinogen with an abnormal structure (e.g. with replacement of a specific amino acid due to a mutation) can also cause a bleeding tendency but is very rare. In these cases there is a prolonged thrombin and/or batroxobin time.

In fibrinolytic (thrombolytic) therapy the fibrinogen level *usually decreases*. In certain situations the therapeutic effect of fibrinolytic therapy can be monitored and evaluated by measuring fibrinogen. Note that the samples must be analyzed without delay so that the fibrinolytic process does not continue and result in a "falsely" low fibrinogen level.

Elevated concentration of fibrinogen in plasma is observed, for example, in an inflammatory reaction (acute phase protein). The elevation lasts longer postoperatively, for instance, than is the case with other acute phase proteins, like C-reactive protein (CRP) and orosomucoid, due to differences in the regulation of biosynthesis and elimination from the blood. An elevated level is also normally seen in *pregnancy*.

An elevated level is associated with an increased risk of myocardial infarction and cerebral thrombosis. Very high levels can be seen in, for example, sepsis. *Note*: Sepsis may be associated with DIC and a single fibrinogen value may be falsely normal in spite of significant consumption. Therefore repeated measurements of fibrinogen concentrations should be made.

Several hereditary mutations that can cause a venous thrombosis are also described.

S-FDP/P-fibrin D-dimer

A marker of hypercoagulation and fibrinolysis, this reflects increased fibrinolytic degradation of increased amounts of intravascular fibrin.

Fibrin D-dimer is primarily *a marker of increased coagulation*. Fibrinolysis is seldom so suppressed that fibrin D-dimer levels are not elevated in connection with an ongoing coagulation activity. Fibrin(ogen) degradation products (FDP) are fibrinolytic products from fibrin as well as fibrinogen. Fibrin D-dimer is a specific degradation product of cross-linked fibrin – an elevated level is present at fibrin formation followed by fibrinolysis. Levels of D-dimer are frequently elevated in medically severely sick patients, post-traumatically and postoperatively, as well as in DIC and in pregnancy toxicosis. High levels of degradation products of fibrin or fibrinogen (e.g. in thrombolytic treatment) inhibit platelet function and can therefore contribute to an increased bleeding tendency. Elevated levels of fibrin D-dimer are also almost always seen in DVT/LE.

The great value of this test in thrombosis diagnosis is the high probability with which a negative test can exclude thrombosis in outpatients, especially in combination with a clinical calculation of probability of the type score-based diagnostic algorithm (compare Wells score) (www.sbu.se). An increased fibrin D-dimer level is, however, more difficult to evaluate and cannot be used to predict the presence of a thrombosis.

Some methods for measuring D-dimer have a relatively high detection limit and do not identify the minor elevations that sometimes occur in a thrombotic disease. Contact your laboratory concerning the detection limit (and the clinical prediction capacity). It is desirable to have a detection level of about 100 µg/L, which is above the upper reference limit in healthy individuals. However, D-dimer methods are poorly standardized and numerical values from different methods can usually not be compared.

Note that the outcome of the test also depends on the examined population, the patient's age, the duration of the thrombosis and its extent. The fibrin D-dimer level is normally elevated (up to twice) during *pregnancy* (see Chapter 12). The level is even more elevated in pre-eclampsia but not so evident in intrauterine growth defect. The level rises with age (for instance, the level is 2–5 times higher in those over 60 years than in younger individuals). In severely ill (hospitalized) patients, the test is of little value for diagnosing thrombosis. The half-life in healthy individuals is normally 15–30 hours.

P-antithrombin

Antithrombin is the most important inhibitor of the coagulation enzymes thrombin and FXa, but also of FXIIa, FXIa and FIXa. Some studies indicate that antithrombin also inhibits kallikrein and plasmin. The physiologic importance of this is not clear.

The activity of antithrombin increases dramatically in the presence of UHF and LMH.

Hereditary deficiency leads to an increased risk of thrombosis. Acquired deficiency, also leading to increased risk of thrombosis, is seen in DIC, sepsis, obstetric complications, heparin treatment for more than 4–5 days, liver damage (antithrombin is synthesized in the liver), malignancy, high-dose estrogen treatment and nephrosis. The level may be slightly elevated during AVK treatment. Antithrombin levels in plasma do not change during a normal pregnancy. However, the level often decreases in pre-eclampsia.

P-anti-Xa analysis to be used in monitoring heparin and LMH treatment

P-heparin or P-LMH-heparin is the earlier name of an assay that is now called anti-factor Xa because several similar anticoagulant drugs can be measured with the same test system. The assay measures the inhibiting effect of UFH, LMH, etc. on FXa. However, in order to obtain relevant values for different LMH, the assay mostly has to be calibrated against the corresponding LMH.

P-heparin/HPF4 for screening of heparin/PF4 antibodies in HIT with ID-PaGIA HPF4 method.

Heparin-induced thrombocytopenia (HIT) is a severe, potentially limb- and life-threatening immune-mediated adverse drug reaction to unfractioned heparin and/or low molecular weight heparin (see Chapter 14). ID-PaGIA HPF4 assay with high-density polymer particles coated with heparin/PF4 complex, which reacts with antibodies in plasma, is a rapid screening method for ruling out HIT diagnosis

Special analyses

Coagulation factors

P-prothrombin (FII), P-factor VII (FVII), P-factor X (FX)

Low levels are mostly found in connection with AVK treatment, liver damage and, in the case of FX, sometimes in amyloidosis. A pronounced hereditary deficiency is very rare for FX and prothrombin but entails a severe bleeding tendency. Hereditary FVII deficiency is somewhat more common but even its severe form seldom leads to bleeding symptoms and does not seem to protect against thrombosis.

P-factor VII and P-factor VII activated

An increased concentration of FVII has been reported to increase the risk of myocardial infarction. The significance of FVII and activated FVII (FVIIa) has, however, not been sufficiently documented.

P-factor V (FV)

Total or partial hereditary FV deficiency is rare. Total deficiency leads to bleeding symptoms similar to those in hemophilia.

P-factor VIII (FVIII)

A low level of FVIII is present in patients with hemophilia type A, carriers of this disease, all patients with severe VWD as well as many with a moderate or mild form.

A consumption-dependent deficiency is often found in DIC with bleeding. FVIII analysis is relatively quick and should be performed in severe bleeding. The possibility of an anticoagulant should be considered if severe bleeding is inexplicable or a prolonged APT time is discovered by chance. These anticoagulants are often turned against FVIII. They should always be assessed when FVIII is low or undetectable in patients who have previously been considered healthy, with no bleeding disorders.

The concentration of FVIII roughly doubles in a normal pregnancy.

The level of FVIII often increases parallel to VWF. An elevated level probably favors coagulation and is associated with an increased risk of DVT/LE. It is also an independent predictor of recurrence. An elevated FVIII level is sometimes inherited but no genetic explanation has been found.

P-factor IX (FIX)

A low FIX level is present in patients with hemophilia type B, in carriers of this disease, and in patients with liver damage, etc. (see above and Chapter 4).

P-factor XI (FXI)

Factor XI deficiency is common in Jews of east European origin. The disorder leads to an increased bleeding risk, above all in surgery, especially oral or of the prostate.

P-factor XII (FXII), P-prokallikrein, P-kininogen

A partial or total deficiency of one of these factors does not lead to an increased bleeding risk. The APT time is moderately to strongly prolonged (in FXII deficiency). Some of these patients may have an increased risk of thrombosis. The disorder needs to be diagnosed in order to avoid an unnecessary investigation of the prolonged APT time and thus delay, e.g. an acute operation.

P-factor XIII (FXIII)

A factor XIII deficiency is occasionally found in patients with a hereditary bleeding disorder. A severe form (total deficiency) often shows symptoms in the neonatal period, such as persistent bleeding from the umbilicus. Spontaneous intracranial bleeding may occur. Decreased fertility and an increased frequency of abortions have been reported in patients with FXIII deficiency. Acquired partial FXIII deficiency has been described in chronic inflammatory intestinal disorders. FXIII is of importance in the healing of wounds.

P-VWF

Von Willebrand factor circulates in the blood in complex with FVIII and can be analyzed as protein/antigen (VWF:Ag) as well as functionally (VWF:RCo or VWF:CB).

VWF is *decreased* in patients with VWD. In severe cases, the factor is only detectable with a sensitive ELISA technique. The ratios FVIII/VWF:Ag and VWF:Ag/VWF:RCo are normally about 1.0. An elevation of FVIII/VWF:Ag ratio is common in mild VWD and can be used as one way of diagnosing the disease, especially if the level is close to the lower reference limit. (The ratio is often decreased, on the other hand, in carriers of hemophilia A and always in mild and moderate forms of hemophilia A and is therefore also useful here for diagnostic purposes.) VWF:Ag/VWF:RCo is usually elevated in type II VWD.

The inter- and intraindividual variations are very large for VWF as well as FVIII and diagnosis can be difficult, especially of mild VWD. As in normal individuals, there is some variation during the menstrual cycle. The best way to diagnose fertile women is to draw samples during the first 4 days of the menstrual cycle. It is, however, most important that the patient arrives at the laboratory in a calm and unrushed state (avoid physical and psychologic stress). A FVIII/VWF quotient of 1.6 or more confirms the diagnosis. However, not all patients with a mild form of the disease have such a quotient. An acquired decreased VWF level is seen, for instance, in certain forms of myeloproliferative diseases.

Elevated VWF levels often appear in inflammatory reactions (acute phase reactant). VWF is synthesized in endothelial cells in the blood vessels. High levels of VWF are therefore a good marker of endothelial damage; levels may be very high in vasculitis, for example. Some studies have found that high concentrations are associated with an increased risk of myocardial infarction. The Leiden Thrombophilia Study indicated that high levels are also a risk factor for DVT/LE. High levels of FVIII and VWF can be seen in liver cirrhosis (the FVIII/VWF:Ag ratio decreases in DIC). Very high levels of VWF in sepsis correlate with a poor prognosis. In a normal pregnancy, VWF concentrations increase about four times. Levels may be very high in pregnancy toxicosis. Measurement of the level can be used to monitor the effects of treatment.

Anticoagulants
P-coagulation surface-induced antibody (screening for coagulation factor inhibitors)

Activated partial thromboplastin (APT) time is measured in different dilutions of patient plasma in normal plasma. The dilution is measured immediately and then after 2 hours of incubation at 37°C. The test requires that the patient's APT time is prolonged at least 5 seconds more than the upper reference level. An APT time that is substantially prolonged in a mixture containing only 10% of the patient's plasma is a strong indication that the patient's plasma contains antibodies which disturb the coagulation process. The antibodies are usually directed against FVIII.

P-factor VIII, antibody

In a test system for measuring FVIII, the dilutions of patient plasma in normal plasma are measured after incubation for 2 hours at 37°C. The result is expressed in Bethesda units. *Note*: the Nijmegen method, which is a modification of the Bethesda method, is more sensitive for low inhibitor titer but is not currently widely used.

P-factor IX, antibody

In a test system for measuring FIX, the dilutions of patient plasma in normal plasma are measured after incubation for 2 hours at 37°C. The result is expressed in Bethesda units.

P-VWF, antibody

In a test system for measuring functional VWF (VWF:RCo), the dilutions of patient plasma in normal plasma are measured after incubation for 2 hours at 37°C.

P-lupus anticoagulant

Thromboembolic manifestations caused by so-called lupus anticoagulants or phospholipid antibodies are seen fairly frequently. These antibodies are directed against phospholipids such as cardiolipin and phosphatidylserine in cell membranes, bound, for example to β2-glycoprotein I. These lupus anticoagulants are developed in pregnancy in particular and secondarily in autoimmune disorders like SLE, rheumatic arthritis, Sjögren's syndrome, and in infectious diseases, above all in bacterial infections; in HIV they occur in 60–80%. The phospholipid antibodies interfere with many coagulation tests and often generate a prolonged APT time. It is not clear how these antibodies interact with the hemostatic system *in vivo* and cause thrombosis formations.

P-, S-cardiolipin antibodies

This test indicates an immunochemical presence of antibodies directed against cardiolipin in plasma or serum. The presence of cardiolipin antibodies does not always lead to a positive lupus anticoagulant result and vice versa.

Protein C anticoagulant system
P-protein S

Protein S is a vitamin K-dependent protein, which is a co-factor to protein C. Protein S in plasma is linked to a considerable extent to the C4b-binding protein. This makes it easy to differentiate between free and total protein S. The free protein S fraction is physiologically active. Hereditary protein S deficiency generates an increased risk of thrombosis. Decreased levels are observed in vitamin K deficiency, liver damage, AVK treatment, DIC and in pregnancy and hormonal treatment (replacement and/or contraceptives). At present, properly standardized methods are available only for detecting free and total protein S antigen. An analysis of free protein S is sufficient to determine whether an individual is sick. Functional methods are being developed.

P-Protein C

Protein C is a vitamin K-dependent coagulation inhibitor. Hereditary protein C deficiency generates an increased risk of thrombosis. An acquired deficiency is observed in connection with vitamin K deficiency, AVK treatment, liver damage and DIC. APC acts among other things through degradation of activated FVIII and FV. In normal pregnancy, protein C increases initially and then decreases.

P-activated protein C resistance = APC resistance

Activated protein C resistance is the most common known reason for a hereditary venous thromboembolic disorder in which APC cannot link to and degrade the mutant form of FVa and it usually depends on a hereditary mutation in the FV gene (1691G>A), named FV Leiden. This defect is present in more than 90% of patients with APC resistance.

Activated protein C resistance can be measured with the original functional method (the ratio of APT time with and without addition of APC) where intraindividual differences between sampling occasions make it necessary to perform confirming assays, for instance in connection with pregnancy or anticoagulant therapy. We now have a more secure method that can be used during AVK and heparin treatment (dilute samples with FV-deficient plasma). APC resistance cannot be determined correctly if the patient's APT time is initially prolonged, as is the case, for instance, in the presence of phospholipid antibodies. Individuals with a so-called acquired APC resistance (no mutation but a positive result of the original APC assay) may also have an increased tendency to thrombosis.

The DNA diagnosis using PCR technique gives a more adequate answer than the conventional measurement of APC resistance. The analysis of mutation 1691G>A cannot, of course, detect an acquired APC resistance. If this is suspected (e.g. in pregnancy), a functional analysis must be performed.

Platelet function

P-platelet aggregation (Pt-agg)

One reason for performing Pt-agg may be a prolonged capillary bleeding time in spite of normal platelet count and VWF levels. Functional platelet defects are the most common hemostatic defects. In the test, ADP, adrenaline, collagen, ristocetin and arachidonic acid are added to the patient's platelets, often making it possible to judge which type of functional defect is present. However, the sensitivity of the test is limited – only severe defects, such as Glanzmann's thromboasthenia and Bernhard–Soulier syndrome, are clearly pathologic.

P-heparin-induced platelet aggregation (HIPA)
This is used in HIT diagnostics. It measures activation of platelets in healthy donor washed platlets after the addition of patient plasma and heparin (concentration 0.1–1 IU/mL). The sensitivity of this method is good (>90%) while the specificity for detecting clinically relevant (pathogenic) antibodies is higher than with commercially available antigen assays (see below) As the assay is sometimes difficult to evaluate, an ELISA test is used as a rule as a primary assay.

P-heparin antibodies ELISA
This detects circulating IgG, IgA and IgM antibodies against heparin/PF4 complex. Since only some antibodies (e.g. IgG) are of clinical importance, sensitivity to all three subclasses of antibodies decreases assay specificity (50–93%). At the same time, the sensitivity of this method is high (>97%) with a negative predictive value of >95%. Therefore negative results obtained with ELISA may be used for ruling out a HIT diagnosis, while positive results should be combined with clinical findings and/or the above functional assay.

Fibrinolysis
P-plasminogen
Hereditary plasminogen deficiency is very rare and is connected with thromboembolic events. An acquired plasminogen deficiency is present in liver disease, often in connection with thrombolytic treatment, and occasionally in DIC.

P-plasmin inhibitor (α2-antiplasmin)
The protein is a weak acute phase reactant. It is often consumed in DIC. Low levels are seen above all in liver diseases and in connection with thrombolytic treatment. Hereditary total deficiency is very rare and, as a result of increased fibrinolysis, leads to a severe bleeding disorder, including muscle and joint bleeding, similar to those in severe hemophilia.

P-plasminogen activator, tissue type (t-PA)
The t-PA, normally present in plasma, is released from the endothelial cells of the vessels. It activates plasminogen to plasmin in the presence of

fibrin. A decreased release of this activator (measured as activity) entails a decreased fibrinolytic capacity. In order to assess the situation, t-PA can be measured before and after a provocation (e.g. venous stasis, 1-desamino-8d-arginine vasopressin (DDAVP) or physical effort). In plasma, the largest component of t-PA, measured as an antigen, consists of an enzymatic inactive complex with PAI-1. An elevated level of the antigen indicates an increased risk of arterial complications, including myocardial infarction. At present, this analysis is not recommended for investigating DVT/LE but can be performed in investigations of arterial thromboembolism. The level increases with age.

P-plasminogen activator-inhibitor-1 (PAI-1) (P-tissue plasminogen activator inhibitor-1)

An increased concentration of PAI-1 causes reduced activity of t-PA and thereby worsens the fibrinolytic function. An elevated concentration of PAI-1 is associated with an increased risk of DVT/LE as well as myocardial infarction. Elevated levels are often seen in obesity, physical inactivity, high levels of blood lipids (especially triglycerides) and in the so-called metabolic syndrome (insulin resistance). PAI-1 is an acute phase reactant, often increasing parallel to CRP. Therefore, high levels are also present in many intensive care patients but often decrease quickly after adequate treatment. High levels inhibit fibrinolytic activity and can possibly contribute to poor "revascularization" of the microcirculation and organ damage. High levels correlate to a poorer prognosis. The level is elevated about five times in pregnancy. PAI-1 levels are often elevated in pre-eclampsia. In severe pre-eclampsia, the increased resistance in the placental circulation is correlated with a further increase in PAI-1.

The diurnal variation is quite large, above all in individuals who are homozygous for the 4G allele in the well-known 4G/5G polymorphism in the promotor region of the PAI-1 gene. The plasma concentration peaks during the second half of the night. Sampling should be done between 7 and 10 am (i.e. as early as possible). This must be remembered when collecting control materials.

Total PAI-1 deficiency has been associated with postoperative bleedings in several studies.

Markers of coagulation activation (hypercoagulation markers)

Also, see under fibrin D-dimer and soluble fibrin.

Activating peptides, general remarks

Peptides, small protein fragments, are released from the proenzyme in the activation of several enzymes in the coagulation and fibrinolytic system.

Their presence is subsequently a good marker of activation. However, their concentrations are low as a rule, they have a very short half-life in the circulation and sampling difficulties lead to elevated values. To date, we know most about fibrinopeptide A (FPA) but determination is complex and sampling has to be faultless. One activating peptide that has proved to be relatively useful is prothrombin fragment 1+2. Peptides split off from FIX and FX have also been described as possible markers/predictors.

P-prothrombin fragment 1+2 (F1+2)
The level is elevated in increased coagulation activation, including DIC. The assay has been used in many studies. The half-life in circulation under normal conditions is 60–90 min.

Note: When TAT complex and F1+2 are used to monitor severely ill patients, higher reference values apply to intensive care patients and pregnant women.

P-thrombin-antithrombin (TAT) complex
Thrombin-antithrombin complex is formed when free thrombin is circulating. Elevated levels have been shown, for example, in DVT/LE and DIC. The method is time-consuming and treatment with antithrombin concentrate containing TAT complex makes the result difficult to evaluate. The half-life in the circulation is normally about 15 minutes.

Note that the upper reference limit for TAT complex and F1+2 increases 2–3 times with age. Problems in sampling often lead to falsely high values.

DNA analyses

All assays are performed in whole blood-leukocyte DNA extraction (B Lkc).

DNA-based diagnosis of hemophilia A and B
The DNA-based diagnosis of hemophilia A and B is used to exclude carriers and identify carrier women, such as mothers, daughters, sisters, aunts and female cousins of the patient with a bleeding disorder, in order to give those with a disposition good genetic advice. The purpose is to offer possibilities of prenatal diagnosis, if the carrier wishes to become or is pregnant. DNA diagnosis is especially important in women who have a son with hemophilia and in daughters of hemophiliacs. The investigation should be performed before a pregnancy, if possible. A DNA diagnosis is often much more reliable than coagulation analysis. In order to confirm that a person is a carrier, it is important to have a blood sample for comparison from a family member with hemophilia or from another relevant relative.

A mutation has been identified in the FVIII gene (inversion mutation in intron 22) causing severe hemophilia. This is found in almost 50% of severely ill hemophiliacs attending the Stockholm Hemophilia Center. These families can now be offered a better direct genetic diagnosis. An inversion mutation in intron 1 has also been described. It is very rare but can be analysed at special coagulation and/or genetic laboratories.

Embryo DNA from a chorionic villus (part of the placenta) biopsy is used in prenatal diagnosis. The investigation is normally performed in pregnancy week 10–11. The procedure is based on coupling analysis (indirect gene diagnosis), in which hereditary variations (DNA polymorphisms) are used to follow the heredity of the diseased (mutant) gene in every family. Southern blot and polymerase chain reaction (PCR) are used in the investigations. The cleavage pattern of a hemophiliac patient in the same family has to be known.

DNA-based diagnosis in VWD
With the help of direct mutation screening at the genetic laboratory in co-operation with the coagulation laboratory, it is possible to identify the mutations in the VWF gene in most patients with severe VWD (type 3). It is possible to verify that this form usually appears when both parents have one mutation each. The patient can be homozygous, i.e. a recipient of the same mutation from both parents, or compound heterozygous, i.e. carry two different mutations, one from each parent. However, international studies have shown that most patients with mild VWD are heterozygous for one mutation in the VWF gene. But even heterozygous individuals can develop a phenotypically severe form. In families where the mutations have been identified, conditions favor a reliable diagnosis and embryonal diagnosis can be performed when desired. In practice, this is not yet a clinical routine.

DNA-based diagnosis in other hereditary bleeding disorders
DNA assays are performed in many laboratories. Information can be obtained from the coagulation units.

DNA-based diagnosis in thromboembolic disorders
Mutation 1691G>A in the factor V gene is known as the Leiden mutation. The frequency of the FV Leiden mutation (1691G>A) is about 5% in Caucasians while it is almost absent in Chinese. In patients with this mutation, the risk of developing DVT/LE is increased about seven times, while for those who are homozygous for this mutation the risk is increased more than 50-fold. This means that many heterozygous individuals will be asymptomatic for the rest of their lives. See also APC resistance.

Mutation 20210G>A in the prothrombin gene
This mutation (polymorphism) is present in about 2% of the normal population and is a weak but independent risk factor for DVT/LE. It leads to slightly elevated levels of prothrombin. The exact mechanism is not yet known.

Mutation analyses – other
Many mutations leading to thromboembolic complications have been identified, e.g. in antithrombin and protein C genes. Consult a coagulation specialist to discuss the possibilities for analyses.

Global hemostatic assays and bedside methods

Endogenous thrombin potential (ETP)
Thrombin generation is measured after the addition of a suitable trigger (tissue factor, phospholipids and calcium) and the amount of generated thrombin is plotted against time to construct a thrombin generation curve (thrombogram), from which additional parameters are calculated, i.e. lag time, peak height, time to peak and the area under the thrombin generation curve – ETP. Both chromogenic and fluorogenic substrate may be used.

Overall hemostatic potential (OHP)
A quick and simple method has been developed in the coagulation research unit, whereby it is possible to determine the total coagulation balance (OHP), hypercoagulation (OCP = overall coagulation potential) and the fibrinolytic potential (OFP = overall fibrinolytic potential) in plasma. For details see He S, *et al. Thromb Res.* 2001; 103: 355–61. This is still only a research analysis which performs in citrated plasma.

Thromboelastography (TEG)/RoTEG
By following the change in elasticity during clot formation with a mechanical detection system, the assay provides data about clot formation and its physical strength and stability, in addition to any dissolution. Recently, a new portable TEG instrument (RoTEG Coagulation Analyzer) was established. The preferred sample is citrated whole blood but plasma can also be used for experimental work.

Fibrin-gel structure
Some small investigations have revealed an abnormally tight fibrin-gel network in young patients with myocardial infarction, in other patients with cardiac artery disorders, in stroke patients and in uncontrolled diabetes. The fibrin network becomes more porous during treatment with

relatively low doses of ASA. So far, this method is only suitable for scientific investigations.

Point-of-care tests (POCT) – also used as a routine

Today, a number of small instruments are available for measuring the concentrations of some parameters on the ward, in outpatient clinics and even at home. These instruments are usually used for APT time and PT(INR). The Coagucheck is such an instrument available for self-testing of PT(INR).

Other bedside methods have been developed for intensive care and surgical departments. Whole blood is normally used. The result is a graphic picture of the coagulation-hemostatic process. The curves can be interpreted to indicate whether or not there is an influence on the primary and/or secondary hemostasis.

Apart from TEG/RoTEG, REOROX and Sonoclot are also used. They are built on different principles and different reagents are used. Systems for controlling reproducibility, etc. are often lacking. Neither is the interpretation always properly standardized and it depends to a great extent on personal experience.

Useful components in research studies

P-soluble fibrin

Soluble fibrin (previously known as fibrin monomers) is an intermediate between fibrinogen and fibrin. Above-normal concentrations are thus a reliable sign of increased fibrin formation in the circulation. The method can be used to diagnose hypercoagulation (even in DIC) and to monitor the effect of treatment of such conditions. The most tested method at present uses a chromogenic substrate to measure the effect of the soluble fibrin on activation of plasminogen with t-PA. There are also immunochemical assays but there is often a cross-reaction with fibrin degradation products. The half-life of soluble fibrin in the circulation is normally 4–6 hours.

P-plasmin-plasmin inhibitor complex

The complex forms upon inactivation of free plasmin. It indicates an ongoing fibrinolytic activation. It is a good predictor of elevated primary and secondary fibrinolysis, particularly useful in promyelocytic leukemia and prostate cancer.

P-t-PA-PAI complex

An increase in this complex is a better marker of DVT/LE, and above all of myocardial infarction, than an increase in t-PA antigen.

P-thrombin time

Thrombin time is prolonged in the presence of heparin (UFH, LMH), high concentrations of fibrinolytic products, low fibrinogen concentrations and hereditary fibrinogen dysfunction.

P-batroxobin time

This analysis has the same range of applications as thrombin time but is not sensitive to the presence of heparin (UFH, LMH).

P-C1-esterase inhibitor

The C1-esterase inhibitor is the only inhibitor of C1-esterase in the complement system, but is also an inhibitor of kallikrein and FXIIa. Consequently the concentration is often decreased in DIC.

P-elastase

Elastase is released from active granulocytes. It degrades, for example, fibrinogen and fibrin into different FDPs, for instance fibrin D-dimer. Thus, the fibrinolytic activity is not always caused by plasmin. Very high levels are often present in DIC, correlating with a poor prognosis. One elastase inhibitor has recently been discovered.

P-heparin co-factor II (HC II)

Heparin co-factor II is a thrombin inhibitor similar to antithrombin, but it inhibits only thrombin, not other coagulation proteases. Dermatan sulfate couples to HC II and therefore its affinity to thrombin increases in the same way as UFH/LMH increases the affinity of antithrombin. HC II is an inhibitor of thrombin in the connective tissue rather than in the circulation. Decreased levels are seen in liver damage, obstetric complications and DIC. Hereditary thromboembolic deficiencies have been described but family studies have yielded conflicting information about such a deficiency. The test is only performed in special cases.

P-plasminogen activator inhibitor 2 (PAI-2)

Plasminogen activator inhibitor 2 is an inhibitor of fibrinolysis that is produced in the placenta and is only present in the blood in pregnancy. The level in the mother is significantly correlated with the function and weight of the placenta, as well as with the growth of the fetus (not correlated with the severity of the pre-eclampsia).

P-protein C inhibitor

The protein C inhibitor is attracting more and more attention, being an inhibitor of APC but also a very important inhibitor of kallikrein. The activity increases in the presence of heparin. The level is decreased in

DIC. (It is also important in male reproduction.) The level decreases in pregnancy.

P-APC-protein C inhibitor (PCI) complex

The protein C system is essential for keeping blood vessels open, free from thrombi. It is activated in any thromboembolic situation. However, a great deal of the formed APC is quickly inhibited by PCI. Complexes of APC-PCI therefore are found in the circulation in thromboembolic situations. An ELISA method for the assay of these complexes has been developed at the clinical chemistry laboratory in Malmö and preliminary studies have shown promising results, i.e. increased levels of APC-PCI have been found in patients with DIC, thromboembolism, pre-eclampsia, etc. The method is expected to become commercially available in the near future.

P-TAFI

Thrombin activatable fibrinolysis inhibitor is an enzyme (also called carboxypeptidase B, R or U) that has been described relatively recently as an inhibitor of fibrinolysis and can be regarded as a link between coagulation and fibrinolysis. The proenzyme is activated by the thrombin/thrombomodulin complex, after which the enzyme splits off the carboxyterminal lysin and arginin residues from the formed fibrin. The fibrin "co-factor" activity, affecting t-PA, disappears, plasmin cannot easily form and thereby fibrinolysis is downregulated. There are large interindividual but no gender differences. TAFI is decreased *in vitro* in hemophilia (does not easily generate thrombin, so fibrinolysis increases). TAFI levels are increased in APC resistance (more thrombin is generated and thereby inhibits fibrinolysis). TAFI is decreased *in vivo* in liver cirrhosis and in DIC. Several studies describe an increase in cardiovascular disorders and stroke (acute phase reactant?).

P-VWF cleaving protease (VWF cleaving protease = ADAMTS-13)

Only the large VWF multimers are active in hemostasis. The size of VWF is regulated by proteolytic degradation of the binding 842Tyr-843Met in the A2 domain of the VWF via a metalloprotease, the proform of which, ADAMTS-13, is normally present in plasma. The importance of the enzyme is reflected in the disease thrombotic thrombocytopenic purpura (TTP), a condition with a deficiency or decreased function of ADAMTS-13, with extra large multimers and microthromboembolic complications. It is possible that the high VWF levels found in patients with a stable ischemic cardiac disorder are due not only to endothelial damage but also to lower ADAMTS-13 activity. The same may be the case in many situations with high VWF levels. In hereditary TTP there is a deficiency of the proenzyme. In noncongenital TTP, the apparent deficiency is due to an inhibitor (IgG) of the protease.

Patients with the hemolytic uremic syndrome (HUS) do not have a severe VWF protease deficiency but antibodies have developed against the protease (see Chapter 14).

Determination of the concentration of ADAMTS-13 is not a routine procedure. It is done only in special laboratories. However, commercial reagents are under development.

P-tissue factor pathway inhibitor (TFPI)

Tissue factor pathway inhibitor is a FXa-dependent inhibitor of the FVIIa tissue factor complex. The importance of TFPI for the development of thromboembolic events and DIC is still rather uncertain.

P-tissue factor (TF)

Tissue factor is exposed in tissue damage, endothelial damage and on or by white blood cells, especially monocytes, in inflammatory reactions. New methods have been developed for the determination of this factor.

Platelet-activating predictors

P-thromboglobulin (β-TG), P-platelet factor 4 (PF4)

These are two platelet-specific peptides stored in the α granules. Strong platelet stimulation is accompanied by release of the content of α granules into the surrounding plasma. When increased intravascular platelet activation leads to platelet aggregation, increased levels of the two substances are found.

Platelet P-selectin (CD62P) or P-soluble P-selectin

P-selectin is a receptor structure in the α granules membrane. Platelet activation and release of the α granules content expose the granule membrane on the platelet surface. This antigen structure can be demonstrated with flow cytometry. Soluble P-selectin is composed of P-selectin which has been cleaved off enzymatically from the membrane or has not been attached to the granule membrane. It is a useful marker of platelet activation.

PLT-fibrinogen, PLT-VWF

Platelet activation involves the activation of receptors on the surface of the platelets which bind to fibrinogen (receptor GP IIb/IIIa) and VWF (receptor GP Ib/IX) respectively. With flow cytometry, fibrinogen and VWF can be detected on the platelet surface as markers of elevated intravascular platelet activation.

Microparticles (MP)

Microparticles are subcellular structures – microvesicles (<1 μm) released from different cells after activation and/or apoptosis. It has been shown that different types of MP are increased in different atherothrombotic diseases. MPs are also associated with inflammation and complement activation. However, there are still some methodologic problems in the standardization of MP determination. Flow cytometry and ELISA seem to be the most appropriate methods for their testing.

Other nonhemostatic variables of importance

P/S-CRP

An elevated level of CRP is an activity marker of inflammatory disease and also helps to distinguish bacterial infection from other infections and inflammatory stages. CRP has proved to be more efficient for this purpose than, for example, sedimentation rate and white blood cell counts, including differential counts. CRP, using a highly sensitive method (hsCRP), has proved to be a powerful predictor of future cardiovascular disease (myocardial infarction and stroke) in both women and men.

The combination of total cholesterol and CRP in the upper quartiles leads to a greatly increased risk of future cardiovascular disorder. A CRP level above 2 mg/L multiplies the risk.

S-cytokines

The most important cytokines to analyze in trauma, infection and sepsis are the interleukins IL-1, IL-6 and TNF-α. These have a number of proinflammatory effects and contribute pathophysiologically in the above-mentioned conditions. They interact with the coagulation system by potentiating the release of tissue factor from monocytes and damaged endothelium.

P-homocysteine

An elevated level of homocysteine in plasma has been described as correlating with venous thrombosis, as well as arterial disorder. However, recent studies have questioned its importance and therefore homocysteine should be considered as a risk marker rather than a cause of disorders. The mechanism may be hereditary or acquired. The most common cause of acquired hyperhomocysteinemia is a deficiency of vitamin B12 or folic acid. Even when folic acid is within the reference range, its supply can partly or totally normalize the level of homocysteine. It is still not clear whether this leads to a decreased risk of venous thrombosis or arterial disorder.

About 5% of the population have a hereditary cause – a homozygous mutation (677C>T) in the methylenetetrahydrofolic reductase gene – the enzyme becomes thermo-unstable. The folate status is critical for whether the mutation will be dominant for cardiovascular morbidity. The risk increases with increasing levels of homocysteine, without any threshold, and is approximately doubled in the upper 20% of the reference interval, comparable with the increasing risk from hypercholesterolemia or smoking. Mild hyperhomocysteinemia interacts additively with conventional risk factors like hypertension, smoking and hypercholesterolemia.

P-thrombomoduline (TM)

A few rare hereditary TM defects have been described but analysis of TM has not yet proved to be of any importance for investigating thromboembolic disorders. On the other hand, increased levels in plasma can be a marker of vasculitis.

P-fibronectin

Fibronectin (previously called cold-insoluble globulin) is a protein produced by endothelial cells, fibroblasts and cells belonging to the reticuloendothelial system. It acts as an extracellular matrix protein and can bind to collagen, heparin, heparan sulfate and fibrin. When coagulation is activated, half of it binds to fibrin. An increase is a marker of vasculitis. In DIC in severely ill intensive care patients, decreasing levels of fibronectin correlate with a poor prognosis. In pregnancy toxicosis, an elevated level appears before clinical signs.

S-lipoprotein (a) (Lp(a)), P-apolipoprotein

Lipoprotein (a) is an independent risk factor for cardiovascular disorders and cerebrovascular ischemic stroke. It forms a complex with apolipoprotein(a) and LDL. The structure is similar to that of plasminogen. High levels of Lp(a) in plasma are linked to premature coronary syndrome and cerebrovascular insult risk.

P-apolipoprotein A1 (ApoA1) and P-apolipoprotein B (ApoB) concentrations can nowadays be measured in most laboratories with sufficient precision for clinical use and at competitive costs. The ratio P-ApoB/P-ApoA1 has been shown to be a superior marker for risk evaluation of cardiovascular events. The ratio performs better than cholesterol/triglycerides and LDL/HDL ratios in large multinational and multiethnic studies. Target ratios are 0.8 for men and 0.7 for women.

Bleeding disorders

PART 2

Hereditary bleeding disorders

CHAPTER 4

Margareta Holmström[1] and Margareta Blombäck[2]

[1]Department of Medicine, Coagulation Unit, Karolinska Institutet; Hematology Centre, Karolinska University Hospital, Solna, Stockholm, Sweden, [2]Department of Molecular Medicine and Surgery, Coagulation Research, Karolinska Institutet; Clinical Chemistry, Karolinska University Hospital, Solna, Stockholm, Sweden

General remarks about hemophilia A and B

Classical hemophilia is a rare disease and occurs in about 14:100,000 men. Hemophilia A is 4–5 times more common than hemophilia B. Hemophilia is classified as severe, moderate or mild, depending on the degree of deficiency of FVIII or FIX. About half or more of the patients have a severe or moderate form. The disease is X-linked, but in half the number of newborns with hemophilia the disease was not previously known in the family. Joint and muscle bleedings are characteristics of the severe form of hemophilia. These bleedings can occur spontaneously or after a minor trauma. Such bleedings are usually very painful. Without adequate treatment, these bleedings cause synovitis, an increased risk of repeated bleedings in the joint and eventually hemophilic arthropathy, with limited mobility and chronic pain. Most elderly men with severe hemophilia have marked functional impairments. Younger patients who have had prophylactic treatment with factor concentrate from an early age usually have good joint and muscle functions. Patients with severe and moderate forms, with or without known heredity, are diagnosed at an early age. Mild forms, above all have bleedings after operation, tooth extraction or major trauma, are often not diagnosed before adulthood.

Essential Guide to Blood Coagulation. By Jovan P. Antovic and Margareta Blombäck
© Blackwell Publishing, ISBN: 9781405196277

Regular controls at a coagulation center are recommended for patients with hemophilia, including those with mild forms. For severe and moderate hemophilia it is recommended that coagulation status and health in general are checked 1–2 times a year. Children are checked by a coagulation competent pediatrician. For milder forms, controls are conducted every 2–3 years.

Specialists in infectious disease, orthopedic surgeons, rheumatologists, dentists, physiotherapists and social workers, all specialized in treating hemophiliacs serve as consultants to the coagulation centers for patients needing their help.

Note that the amount of coagulation factors is now expressed in international units (kIU/L) or in units per mL (U/mL). The former is used by laboratories that have adopted an international standard. Previously the amount was expressed as a percentage: **100% indicated a normal level and is equivalent to 1 kIU/L or 1 U/mL**.

* **Hemophilia A** – FVIII deficiency
– *severe* form: less than 0.01 U/mL FVIII
– *moderate* form: 0.01–0.05 U/mL FVIII
– *mild* form: 0.06–0.40 U/mL FVIII.

* **Hemophilia B** – FIX deficiency
– *severe* form: less than 0.01 U/mL FIX
– *moderate* form: 0.01–0.05 U/mL FIX
– *mild* form: 0.06–0.40 U/mL FIX

General remarks about von Willebrand's disease

Von Willebrand's disease (VWD) is caused by a quantitative or a qualitative deficiency of Von Willebrand Factor (VWF) that entails a primary hemostatic defect with bleeding symptoms, above all from mucous membranes. A mild form of VWD is the most common type of hereditary bleeding tendency, occurring in about 1% (or less depending on the criteria used). Severe forms are rare, but can cause serious bleeding symptoms resembling those in severe hemophilia. VWD is inherited autosomally, i.e. it occurs in both men and women.

VWD is subdivided into three main types:

Type 1 (earlier type I) is a quantitative defect with a decreased level of VWF, which in other respects is normally structured (normal multimeric pattern); the level of FVIII can be decreased as well. These are mild to moderate forms of VWD. The patients are probably heterozygous with regard to a defect gene. The ratio FVIII/VWF levels is usually high.

Type 2 (earlier type II), comprises all qualitative defects of VWF that cause bleeding symptoms. FVIII may be normal or decreased. Most patients have an abnormal multimeric pattern of the VWF and may be either homozygous or heterozygous with respect to a defect gene. About 20 subtypes have been identified. VWD type 2A lacks the largest multimers. In VWD type 2B, the VWF often has a heightened affinity to platelets, which leads to aggregation and thrombocytopenia. Type 2N lacks the ability to bind FVIII, which means that levels of FVIII are very low and may therefore lead to the false diagnosis of hemophilia A.

Type 3 (earlier type III) patients have no or very low plasma levels of VWF. These patients are severely ill. As a consequence of the low levels of VWF, levels of FVIII are also low because VWF carries FVIII in the circulation. No multimers can be detected.

von Willebrand's disease (VWD) – VWF deficiency
Approximate classification
- *severe* form type 3 (earlier III): VWF less than 0.05 U/mL, FVIII less than 0.10 U/mL, bleeding time prolonged (more than 10 min.)
- *moderate* form: VWF 0.05–0.2 U/mL, FVIII decreased, bleeding time prolonged.
- *mild* form: VWF 0.2–0.5 U/mL, FVIII often somewhat decreased, bleeding time prolonged or normal.

Values were previously expressed as a percentage; 100% indicated a normal level and is equivalent to 1 kIU/L or 1 U/mL.

Factor concentrates used for treatment of hemophilia A and B and VWD in Sweden in 2009

Hemophilia A Factor VIII concentrate
Advate (Baxter)*, Helixate NexGen (CSL Behring)*, Immunate (Baxter), Kogenate-Bayer (Bayer)*, Octanate (Octapharma), Recombinate (Baxter)*, ReFactoAF/Xyntha (Genetics/Wyeth/Lederle)*
* Concentrates developed with biotechnology, using recombinant technique. The others are produced from plasma.

Factor VIII concentrate: In the patient, the yield of the FVIII activity in the concentrate is about 100%.

1 IU FVIII/kg bodyweight increases the plasma concentration by 0.02 IU/mL. The half-life of FVIII is normally 10–14 hours in adults (6–10 hours in children under 5 years). *Note* that in trauma, serious infection, sepsis, when the patient is bleeding and after surgery the half-life may be very short: 2–4 hours.

Example: For serious bleeding in a patient with severe hemophilia, 70 kg bodyweight and a desired FVIII level of 1.00 IU/mL, give $50 \times 70 = 3500$ IU.

Hemophilia B Factor IX concentrate
BeneFIX (Wyeth)*, Immunine (Baxter), Mononine (CSL Behring), Nanotiv (Octapharma).
* Concentrate developed with biotechnology, using recombinant technique.

Factor IX concentrate: The yield in the patient is normally only about 60% (the remaining amount is distributed extravasally), so *1 IU FIX/kg bodyweight increases the plasma concentration by about 0.01 IU/mL.*

The half-life is usually close to 24 hours (shorter for children). A plasma concentration of FIX in the lower part of the treatment areas proposed is mostly sufficient for hemostasis. *Note* that, as with FVIII, the half-life is shorter in trauma, serious infection, sepsis, when the patient is bleeding and after surgery.

Example: For moderate bleeding in a patient with severe hemophilia B, bodyweight 70 kg, and a desired FIX level of 0.5 U/mL, give 3500 IU FIX.

Von Willebrand's disease Factor concentrates with VWF 2008:
Haemate (CSL Behring)
Wilate (Octapharma).

General remarks about factor concentrates
The appropriate concentrate for each patient is chosen by doctors at the coagulation center. Never alter the treatment without consulting the patient's regular center.

As n*ew concentrates are introduced from time to time and current products are constantly reassessed, a coagulation expert (coagulation unit) should be consulted frequently for prescription and advice concerning factor concentrates.*

All factor concentrates approved today are now virus-inactivated with at least one method: chemical additives and/or moist-heat treatment. Furthermore, blood/plasma donors are checked at every donation for *HIV antibodies, HbsAg, hepatitis C antibodies* and often for increase of *transaminases,* and many plasma pools/concentrates are checked for hepatitis viruses with PCR technique. This has eliminated the risk of HIV infection and substantially reduced the risk of hepatitis infection. Patients who have not been treated before usually get recombinant factor concentrates.

Current inactivation methods eliminate enveloped viruses in particular. Non-enveloped viruses, e.g. parvovirus and hepatitis A virus, have been detected in plasma-derived concentrates.

Treatment strategy in severe forms of hemophilia and VWD

Home/self-treatment

Many patients with severe or moderate hemophilia have learned how to administer factor concentrate intravenously themselves at home. Advice concerning treatment and dosage of the concentrates can be obtained from the coagulation unit. Persons treated as out-patients or at the emergency unit are requested to bring their own concentrates, if possible.

Treatment in trauma and acute bleedings

Patients with severe forms of hemophilia and VWD run a high risk of mortality and morbidity if adequate treatment with factor concentrates is not given for bleedings or trauma. Treatment with plasma is not sufficient. If nothing else is available, however, treatment for a serious bleeding or trauma can start with fresh or fresh frozen plasma and tranexamic acid, pending rapid delivery of concentrate.

In the event of an **accident, head trauma, abdominal trauma** or **gastrointestinal bleeding,** patients are instructed to go to a hospital. **Immediate treatment** with factor concentrates in these cases is usually **urgent** and should begin, if possible, at home or at the site of the accident. **The coagulation doctor on duty should always be contacted immediately.**

The bleedings etc. listed below are regarded as severe and should be treated *immediately* with factor concentrate:

FVIII concentrate 40–50 IU/kg bodyweight or *FIX concentrate 70–80 IU/kg bodyweight.*

Important rules etc. for initial treatment with factor concentrates

The requisite amount of factor concentrate is calculated from

* desired level in plasma (U/mL)

* bodyweight (kg)

The calculated volume is rounded up to the nearest whole bottle or ampoule.

[If B-EVF (hematocrit) is low, correct the volume upwards if erythrocyte concentrate is not given.]

RECOMMENDATIONS FOR DESIRED INITIAL PLASMA CONCENTRATIONS AT DIFFERENT TYPES OF BLEEDINGS

A single treatment is not sufficient in more severe forms of hemophilia and should be repeated in relation to the magnitude of the trauma for several days or longer (weeks?). **About further treatment, contact the coagulation doctor on duty.**

- **Head trauma, abdominal trauma, severe external injury, suspected retroperitoneal bleeding**

Desired initial plasma concentration 0.8–1.2 U/mL.
Trauma to the head *may cause intracranial bleeding even in* **mild forms** *of bleeding disorders.*
Neurological signs at head trauma do not in general show initially; they may appear after several days or even weeks.

- **Gastrointestinal bleeding**
  Desired initial plasma concentration minor 0.4–0.6 U/mL
  severe 0.8–1.2 U/mL
- **Suspected bleeding in the throat and face region**
  Desired initial plasma concentration: 0.8–1.2 U/mL
- **Muscle bleedings in iliopsoas**
  Risk of compression of the femoral nerve. Immobilization and a high leg position initially are recommended.
  Desired initial plasma concentration 0.8–1.2 U/mL
- **Muscle bleeding in the calf or lower arm**
  Risk of compartment syndrome.
  Desired initial plasma concentration: 0.8–1.2 U/mL
- **Joint and other types of muscle bleedings**
  SYMPTOMS AT JOINT AND MUSCLE BLEEDINGS

	Minor	*Moderate*	*Severe*
Pain	+/–	+	++
Swelling	–	(+)	+
Restricted movement	(+)	+	++
Nerve involvement	–	–	+

The symptoms of minor joint bleeding can be a pricking or creeping feeling of discomfort that remains or gets worse. "Trust the patient!" A serious joint bleeding can be extremely painful.

In addition to treatment with factor concentrate, we recommend resting the affected leg. Cooling can have a favourable effect on bleeding and pain.

Desired initial plasma concentration:
minor symptoms 0.3 U/mL
moderate symptoms 0.4 U/mL
severe symptoms 0.6–0.8 U/mL

Maintenance treatment
- Minor bleeding: continue conventional prophylaxis (see below)
- Otherwise: give 20–40 IU/kg bodyweight once/24 hours (possibly twice/24 hours in hemophilia A) for 2–6 days, depending on the degree of bleeding, or until there is no discomfort. Always contact the coagulation unit for advice.

Conventional prophylaxis thereafter. For severe joint bleeding with remaining synovitis or repeated bleeding symptoms, increase the intensity of the prophylaxis.

All patients with moderate to severe forms of hemophilia are provided with an individual care plan containing personally calculated instructions as to dosage and intervals for different types of bleeding.

Prophylaxis against joint bleedings

In most patients with a severe form of hemophilia, regular prophylactic treatment with factor concentrate begins at 1–2 years of age. *Usually* 20–40 IU/kg bodyweight is given initially once a week. The frequency is increased as soon as possible to twice/week (hemophilia B) or 3–4 times/week (hemophilia A). Similar principles apply to **severe forms of** VWD.

Bleeding prophylaxis is maintained during the growing period, after which some patients continue with regular prophylaxis while others turn to "on-demand treatment", depending on the frequency and intensity of the bleeding symptoms. As a result of this treatment, most patients with severe hemophilia now reach adult age without damage to joints and muscles.

Physiotherapy is recommended for patients with severe forms in order to prevent invalidity after bleedings and further immobilization in those who already have joint damage.

Regular exercise of various kinds (gymnastics, swimming and other sports) is important, even for those with intact joints, in order to maintain good muscle strength and good coordination. Physical training is coordinated with treatment with factor concentrate. Patients in good physical condition also have a better mental balance.

Home treatment has also reduced the need for hospital care and permitted a significantly better life.

Other important issues

Tranexamic acid (Cyklokapron). Treatment with factor concentrate is often combined with tranexamic acid treatment, especially for joint and muscle bleedings. The dosage is 20 mg/kg bodyweight × 3 perorally or 10 mg/kg i.v. × 3.

Surgery in patients with bleeding disorders

Both major elective surgery and minor surgery with a high risk of bleeding **shall** *be performed in a hospital with a coagulation laboratory and a coagulation unit.*

Daily contact *with the coagulation doctor on duty is also important in every case!*

Remember that surgery always has to be preceded by prophylactic treatment with factor concentrate (or with desmopressin in special mild cases of VWD). A schedule shall be drawn up in cooperation with the coagulation unit at least one week prior to a planned operation. It is important that the schedule is followed in every respect. After the surgery, the patient **shall** be monitored with analyses of the factor that he/she is lacking because the in vivo consumption of factors varies between individuals and between different kinds of surgery. It follows that the schedule may need to be adjusted. For half-lives, see Factor VIII, Factor IX and Von Willebrand factor.

Tooth extraction in a hemophilia patient

is conducted in cooperation with a coagulation unit and its consulting dentist. Prior to the extraction, treatment with factor concentrate should be given as well as tranexamic acid (Cyklokapron) both locally as a mouth wash and on the scar and orally, which reduces the need of hemostatic factor concentrates.

Mild hemophilia patients (i.e. not severe or moderate hemophilia A/ hemophilia B/VWD or a serious platelet function disorder) only need to use a mouth wash, possibly in combination with desmopressin (not active in hemophilia B).

Caution in patients with bleeding disorders

- **High blood pressure combined with bleeding disorders can cause hemorrhage of the brain.** Monitor blood pressure continuously in severe hemophilia/VWD/defective platelet function. *The same applies to patients with moderate and, in many cases, mild forms.*
  If blood pressure is high, it should be treated without delay.
- **Arterial punctures and intramuscular injections should be avoided.**
- **Epidural/spinal anesthesia should not be given to patients with bleeding disorders.**
- **Do not take blood samples from the femoral vein in small children** with a suspected bleeding disorder.
- **Bleeding after a vein puncture** is stopped by compression until the bleeding is brought to a standstill.
- **Drugs** containing *ASA (acetylsalicylic acid)*, long-term *NSAID* drugs, dextran and heparin (UFH and LMH) and thrombin inhibitors can cause serious/life-threatening bleeding in more severe bleeding disorders.

Pain-killing drugs allowed in hemophilia
Analgesics (pain killers)
Pain killers: paracetamol (Alvedon, Panodil), codein (Citodon), dextro-propoxifen (Doloxene, Dexofen), and possibly morphine, petidin etc.

do not increase the risk of bleeding. The morphine group of analgesics should be prescribed with caution in view of the risk of addiction.

Anti-flogistics (against inflammation)

Treatment should be planned together with a coagulation expert. With *clear indications*, anti-inflammatory drugs with a short half-life (ibuprofen, diclofenac) can be given even to severely ill patients with bleeding disorders for long term treatment. COX-2-inhibitors (Celebra, Arcoxia) do not affect platelet function and are especially adequate for patients with chronic synovitis for short term treatment. At present (2009) however, the Swedish Medical Products Agency warns against long-term treatment with these drugs.

Side-effects, primarily in more severe forms of hemophilia and VWD

Anticoagulants

Always contact the coagulation unit.

If treatment with factor concentrates does not have the expected effect, it should be followed by taking samples before and after treatment to determine the level of the factor in question and the presence of anticoagulants, i.e. antibodies against the coagulation factor that is deficient in the patient. Antibodies develop after a varied number of treatments (usually <50) in 15–20% of patients with the more severe forms of hemophilia A and in 2–5% of those with hemophilia B. Patients with VWD may develop antibodies, too. In the above cases, the inhibitors have to be neutralized with concentrate before a desired hemostatic concentration is obtained. This is not possible at high levels of antibodies. Activated concentrates, such as Feiba (Baxter), are used for patients with hemophilia A.

Another form of treatment for these patients is the elimination of antibodies by means of a daily supply of a high dose of the deficient factor (so called immune tolerance treatment). Moreover, treatment with recombinant FVIIa (Novo Seven, Novo Nordisk) has been shown to stop severe bleedings, including joint bleedings, irrespective of the level of anti-bodies. It is also useful in surgery. rVIIa can be used both in hemophilia A and hemophilia B.

Risk of hepatitis

Patients with bleeding disorders are recommended vaccination against hepatitis A and B if future treatment with blood products/factor concentrates is expected.

Antibodies against hepatitis C are present as a consequence of treatment with factor concentrates and/or plasma in up to 90% of adult patients with severe or moderate hemophilia, as well as in some elderly patients with mild hemophilia. Moreover, many patients developed anti-bodies against hepatitis B before vaccination was introduced. Most of the patients with hepatitis C antibodies have intermittently increased levels of transaminases and a chronic hepatitis C infection. Some have suffered/suffer from serious late complications, such as liver cirrhosis and hepatic-cellular cancer. Liver transplantation has been performed in recent years to save life and this has simultaneously cured hemophilia A as well as B. A current treatment for hepatitis C, effective in about 60% of the patients, is pegylated interferon and ribavirin.

Treatment principles for different types of bleeding disorders (severe, moderate and milder forms of hemostatic defects)

Hematuria

Withdraw treatment with tranexamic acid (Cyklokapron, Tranon).

Minor hematuria: Prednisolon 0.5 mg/kg bodyweight/24 hours for 5 days, followed by 0.25 mg/kg bodyweight/24 hours for 5 days can be considered. Copious fluid intake.

Massive hematuria: Possibly factor concentrate in order to obtain a factor level of about 0.3 U/mL. As much rest as possible. Copious fluid intake. Contact the coagulation doctor on duty for advice.

For patients with *mild* hemophilia A or VWD: try desmopressin (see below).

Nose bleeding

Usual local measures, e.g. blood-stilling cotton and mucous membrane softeners. Give tranexamic acid (Cyklokapron). For persistent bleeding, give factor concentrate (for patients with *severe or moderate hemophilia and VWD*) and contact the coagulation doctor on duty.

Experience shows that etching and similar measures should be used very restrictively. Laser treatment can be a more adequate alternative for recurrent bleeding.

For patients with *mild* hemophilia A or VWD, try desmopressin (see below).

Gum bleeding

Gum bleedings is often caused by poor oral hygiene and associated gingi-vitis. Local treatment and control by a dentist or dental hygienist. Mouth wash with solution of tranexamic acid (the onr usually used for iv injection Mix Cyklokapron (100 mg/mL) 5 mL with 5 mL distilled water. Rinse for 1–2 minutes every 8th hour or when needed-helps to reduce bleeding. Ordinary mouth wash can also be used. Also see the end of this manual.

Menorrhagia

Tranexamic acid (Cyklokapron) and/or peroral contraceptives. Access to oral contraceptives has saved the lives of many patients with VWD. Factor concentrates may be needed in more serious cases. For demopressin which is not helpful in neither severe VWD type 3 or in VWD type 2B, see below.

Pregnancy and delivery

Contact a coagulation doctor in order to plan bleeding prophylaxis well in advance. FVIII and VWF increase during the latter part of pregnancy. In patients with mild VWD and hemophilia A carriers, levels are usually normal during the last trimester. This should be verified, preferably after week 32. Patients with more severe VWD may need several weeks of treatment with concentrate after delivery. Epidural-spinal anesthesia cannot be used, due to the risk of bleeding.

Vaginal delivery is recommended, but avoid vacuum and forceps in cases with a known heredity. Umbilical cord blood is often used to diagnose a factor deficiency in cases with known heredity.

Treatment with tranexamic acid – Cyklokapron, Tranon (the latter only available as tablets)

These fibrinolysis inhibitors are often effective in mild, moderate and severe hemophilia patients (most often as an additional treatment), as well as in all patients with VWD or with platelet function defects. They are useful in: mucous membrane bleedings, nose bleedings, gum bleedings, intestinal bleedings, in menorrhagia, in other bleedings, at tooth extractions and surgery. In mild forms of hemophilia A, VWD or thrombocytopathia they are often combined with desmopressin (DDAVP), and with factor concentrate treatment in more severe bleeding disorders. Dosage: Injection of. tranexamic acid (Cyklokapron 10 mg/kg bodyweight iv) or mixture 20 mg/kg bodyweight orally every 8th hour. In Sweden the drug can also be purchased in tablet form (Cyklo-F) without a prescription. The mixture is sold under the name Tranexamic acid as an ex-tempore preparation. See the end of this manual.

Contraindication

Macroscopic hematuria is an important contraindication to tranexamic acid (Cyklokapron, Tranon due to the risk of urethral clotting and thus a possible hydronephrosis).

Severe platelet function defect, e.g. Glanzmann's thrombastenia

This is a rare disorder. Note that most of the principles for treatment that have been outlined above should also be observed in this disease. However, FVIII or FIX concentrates are of no use in these patients, who during childhood display a pronounced tendency to mucous membrane bleedings and hematomas. The diagnosis is confirmed by a markedly prolonged bleeding time and by studying receptors and platelet aggregation capacity. Severe forms of platelet function defect with little or no response to desmopressin treatment should be handled in consultation with a coagulation expert. In acute bleeding situations these patients are primarily treated with leucocyte-filtered platelet (in order to reduce the risk of platelet antibodies) concentrates in combination with tranexamic acid (except in hematuria). However, there is a risk that repeated treatments with desmopressin lead to the development of platelet antibodies, so such treatment should be restricted to clear indications. Recombinant factor VIIa (Novo Seven, Novo Nordisk) has resulted in effective hemostasis in a number of cases and is licensed in Europe for use in patients with Glanzmanns disease.

Mild hemostatic defects

General remarks

Bleeding disorders in a mild form are found in 3–5% of the population in several countries, usually a mild form of von Willebrand's disease (VWD), or a mild platelet function disorder, causing an increased bleeding tendency. These hemostatic disorders are characterised by mucous membrane bleedings and spontaneous bruises, whereas joint and muscle bleedings are rare. Examples are persons with bleeding troubles in connection with an intake of acetylsalicylic acid (ASA) or NSAID, postoperative bleedings and bleeding after a tooth extraction, with no surgical explanation for the bleeding. Such disorders are also present in persons with frequent nose-bleedings, gastrointestinal bleeding or menorrhagia, where no pathologic anatomic explanation can be found. Brain haemorrhage can however also develop in such patients.

Treatment (general)
- *First and foremost, give the patient accurate information.*
- The patient shall avoid ASA and anti-phlogistic drugs.

The risk of intra-cerebral bleeding after a head trauma or in connection with high blood pressure in milder forms of bleeding disorders does not seem to have been studied scientifically. However, there are reasons for being observant.

- Patients with milder hemostatic disorders are investigated in the coagulation unit and then often return to their regular doctor, who contacts the coagulation unit when necessary.

Treatment with desmopressin (Octostim®)

Desmopressin induces endothelial cell release of VWF and FVIII and can improve the interaction between defective platelets and the vessel wall. Desmopressin is therefore effective at various bleedings in patients with *type 1 VWD* and in *primary or secondary platelet function defects* and in mild hemophilia A. Treatment with desmopressin should almost always be combined with tranexamic acid (except in hematuria).

Desmopressin has no effect in

- *Severe deficiency of VWF or FVIII (VWD type 3 and severe hemophilia A)*, as neither VWF nor FVIII is stored in the endothelium in these patients.
- *The serious platelet function defect thrombasthenia Glanzmann.*
- *In VWD type IIb, Desmopressin can induce thrombocytopenia, in which case no hemostatic effect is obtained.*

If the patient fails to respond to the treatment, contact the coagulation unit.

Desmopressin, Octostim® 15 µg/mL (Ferring), is a synthetically produced peptide, modified according to the natural anti-diuretic hormone ADH.

Octostim 0.3 µg/kg bodyweight iv increases the plasma levels of VWF and FVIII 2–3 times resulting in a well documented effective treatment of *mild forms of VWD and hemophilia A* (FVIII deficiency), including carriers of this disease. Octostim may also have some effect in moderate forms of these diseases, but is often then insufficient for good hemostasis.

The effect of desmopressin should be tested prior to planned surgery. The intraindividual response is relatively constant, but 10% do not respond with improved hemostasis and a shortening of the bleeding time. Responders to the treatment (cause unknown) cannot be identified in advance.

For such an investigation, desmopressin (Octostim®) is usually given at 0.2–0.3 µg/kg bodyweight subcutaneously near the umbilicus, with control of the bleeding time after 1 hour.

For treatment desmopressin is usually given subcutaneously and in some cases intravenously; dose Octostim® 0.2–0.3 µg/kg bodyweight (see manufacturer instructions).

Desmopressin (Octostim®) can also sometimes be administrated as a nasal spray, 150 microgram per dose, e.g. in *menorrhagia* in patients with mild VWD or with a platelet function defect. In these cases it is mostly combined with tranexamic acid.

Desmopressin treatment can be repeated if necessary after 6–12 hours. *Note that desmopressin can cause FLUID retention, which can be treated with furosemid according to need.* See below.

Contraindications and side-effects of desmopressin

Desmopressin (Octostim®) **is not recommended** in patients with *an untreated hypertension, unstable angina* or *after a myocardial infection.*

In all patients and especially in *young children* and *pregnant women*, the risk of fluid retention and hyponatriemia should be considered, especially at repeated doses. Seizures are associated with desmopressin treatment and desmopressin should be used with great caution in children under two years of age.

With repeated doses of desmopressin, the fluid balance and S-Na+ should always be monitored, regardless of the patient's age, and only isotonic fluids may be used.

Blood sampling in bleeding disorders

Note the following when sampling blood from patients with bleeding disorders.

Most of the patients who have been treated with blood products have had hepatitis B, and many, including some teenagers, have a chronic hepatitis C. Moreover, some adults have been exposed to HIV contamination through treatment with concentrate. *Follow the rules from your hospital's hygiene committee concerning blood sampling, identification of tubes, etc.*

BLEEDING RISK
INCREASED BLEEDING TENDENCY

Space for photo

BIRTH DATE
or Soc. Security Number

Name and Surname

Physician in charge:

Valid until: 2014-

Coagulation clinic Karolinska University Hospital Solna 171 76 Stockholm Tel +46 8 517 700 00	Coagulation clinic University Hospital MAS 205 02 Malmö Tel +46 40 33 10 00	Coagulation center SU/Sahlgrenska 413 45 Gothenburg Tel +46 31 342 10 00

Front side of a risk chart for anyone with a risk of bleeding.

Bleeding risk charts

Individuals in whom a hereditary bleeding disorder has been diagnosed are requested to wear a bleeding risk chart. These charts are individually designed and differ between coagulation centers.

```
Kortinnehavaren     CAVE              NNNNN MMMMMM
NNNN  MMMMMM        •Aspirin          has an increased
123456-7890         •NSAID            bleeding
har ökad            •Dextran          tendency,
blödnings-          •Intramuscular    von Willebrands
benägenhet p.g.a     injection        disease with a
von Willebrands                       plasma vW factor
sjukdom med vW-                       level of
faktor halt i                         _ XX % and
plasma              Intolerance       should, in case
_ XX % och ska      to:               of accident, all
vid olycksfall,     . . . . . . . . . . . .    head injuries,
skall-skador,       . . . . . . . . . . . .    haemorr-hage and
blödningar, och     . . . . . . . . . . . .    before surgery,
inför kirurgi       . . . . . . . . . . . .    be treated with
erhål-la:           . . . . . . . . . . . .    DDAVP and/or vW-
Octostim och /      . . . . . . .              factor
eller vW-                              concentrate +
faktorkoncentrat                      tranexamic acid.
+ Cyklokapron.                        A doctor on duty
Kontakta i dessa                      for haemostasis
fall alltid                           should always be
koagulationsjour                      contacted.
```

Factor concentrates can be obtained from Apoteket CW Scheele; 08-4548100.

Reverse side of a risk chart for a moderate or mild form of Von Willebrand's disease

Critical bleedings

CHAPTER 5

Hans Johnsson

Department of Emergency Medicine, Karolinska Institutet; Karolinska
University Hospital, Solna, Stockholm, Sweden

Introduction

Serious bleeding implies massive bleeding or a threat to a vital organ,
such as the brain, the throat or a muscle with threatening compartment
syndromes.

Serious bleeding needs to be identified at an early stage to take action
against causes and hemostatic failure. This involves trying to localize
and treat an active bleeding source, low platelet function, consumption
of coagulation factors and increased fibrinolysis. The longer it takes to get
the bleeding under control, the more the whole coagulation process will
be affected.

Bleeding might be aggravated by kidney and liver failure, malignancy
or ongoing treatment with anticoagulant and platelet inhibitory drugs.

Massive bleeding

A massive bleeding is usually defined in terms of blood loss during a certain period of time, numbers of erythrocyte concentrates given to replace
the loss and whether the bleeding reoccurs within a certain period of time.

- Replacement of one blood volume within 24 hours.
- Transfusion of more than four erythrocyte concentrates within an hour
  and when bleeding continues.
- Replacement of more than 50% of the blood volume within 3 hours.
- One unit of erythrocyte concentrate per 10 kg bodyweight per hour and
  still bleeding.

Essential Guide to Blood Coagulation. By Jovan P. Antovic and Margareta Blombäck
© Blackwell Publishing, ISBN: 9781405196277

Massive bleeding may cause the platelet concentration to drop more than 50%, PT(INR) may rise above 1.5 and fibrinogen concentration may drop below 1 g/L. The APT time usually is prolonged to more than 1.5 times the upper reference value, indicating that the concentrations of isolated coagulation factors have dropped to below 30–40% of the reference levels. These changes signify that the coagulation factors and platelet counts have dropped to levels that are critical for adequate hemostasis.

Transfusion coagulopathy

In massive bleeding that requires blood transfusion, several factors are important for the development of transfusion coagulopathy with diffuse microvascular oozing of blood.

- Inhibited synthesis of coagulation factors in the liver and of platelets in the bone marrow.
- Dilution, consumption and proteolysis of platelets and coagulation factors.
- Disturbances in the coagulation process due to citrate-induced hypocalcemia.
- Hypothermia. (<36°C).
- Acidosis. (pH <7.2)
- Low hematocrit (<30%).

Treatment

General procedures

- *Keep the patient warm.* Body temperature below 36°C impairs hemostasis. The platelet function deteriorates, coagulation process is slowed and fibrinolytic activity will increase. This calls for preheated infusion solutions, a warm room and covering the patient with warm blankets or similar.
- *Try to raise hematocrit above 30%.* A low hematocrit alters the flow conditions (shear rate) in small vessels and capillaries. The platelets no longer circulate in a laminar layer just beneath and in close contact with the endothelium, leading to impaired capillary hemostasis.
- *Correct acidosis and hypocalcemia.* A decreasing pH impairs platelet function and the coagulation process. A pronounced hemostatic dysfunction is observed at a pH below 7.2 and at free calcium concentrations below 1 mmol/L.
- *Keep the patient calm and free from pain,* Pain and anxiety are stress factors that impair the body's hemostatic capacity.

In the acute phase, take samples for PT(INR), platelet count, APT time and fibrinogen. There is no universal test for measuring hemostasis but bedside instruments may be useful for a quick estimate, e.g. PT(INR), TEG/ROTEG, etc. Do not wait for laboratory results before starting treatment with:

- plasma, 15–30 mL/kg bodyweight
- platelet concentrate, two units to an adult.

Consider substitution with fibrinogen concentrate.

The aims in continuous bleeding are to maintain:

- Platelet count above $50-100 \times 10^9/L$
- PT(INR) below 1.5
- APT time shorter than 1.5 times the reference value
- fibrinogen above 2 g/L.

Note that treatment with synthetic colloids can give falsely high fibrinogen levels. In these cases, aim for a fibrinogen level above 2.5 g/L.

Choice of plasma

Some blood centers supply both fresh-stored (not more than 2 weeks in a refrigerator) and fresh-frozen plasma. Defrosting the fresh-frozen plasma takes rather a long time, about 45 minutes. In an acute situation the fresh-stored plasma is preferable; its concentrations of the most important coagulation factors are only slightly lower than those in fresh-frozen plasma.

Local procedures

Patients in acute hypovolemic shock due to bleeding, in whom the shock cannot be corrected or reoccurs soon after the initial treatment, often require acute surgery regardless of any hemostatic disturbance.

An early examination of the possibilities of endovascular treatment is important for the prognosis. It can be done with selective embolization or thrombotizing (Spongostan, particles, coils or tissue paste), vasoconstrictive drugs (vasopressin) or covered stents. Such stents are also used in rupturing aneurysm of the aorta and other major vessels.

Angiography also provides an opportunity of stabilizing the circulation with an occluding aorta balloon and creating a respite for other actions.

Additional treatment

In certain situations, treatment with plasma and platelet concentrate is not sufficient to achieve full hemostasis and normalize coagulation.

Fibrinogen concentrate

Fibrinogen concentrates are available on general license at blood centers and hospital pharmacies. Dry ampoules contain 1 g of fibrinogen, and the outcome after administration is about 85%. In an adult weighing 70 kg with an expected plasma volume of 3 L, 1 g of fibrinogen increases the concentration of fibrinogen by 0.3 g/L.

Prothrombin-complex concentrate

Prothrombin-complex concentrate contains coagulation factors II, VII, IX, X, protein C and protein S. The concentrates can be used if plasma treatment fails to have a sufficient effect on PT(INR), and in situations where a volume burden with plasma should be avoided in order to reverse a high PT(INR). This may be the case in patients with an excessive consumption of coagulation factors, patients with liver failure or patients being treated with vitamin K antagonists.

For dose and reversal of high PT(INR), see Chapter 8.

Recombinant factor VIIa (NovoSeven)

Recombinant factor VIIa (rVIIa) is a prohemostatic drug containing coagulation factor VII in active form. NovoSeven accelerates platelet activation and thrombin formation locally on an injured vessel. NovoSeven has a short half-life of 2–3 hours, and a clearance corresponding to 30–35 mL/min. In children under 10 years of age the half-life may be shorter and clearance faster.

The use of recombinant VIIa has been associated with thromboembolic complications, mainly when it is used in the absence of an approved recommendation. Controlled studies are needed. The risk of complications has to be weighed against the expected benefit in the individual situation.

There are still no conclusive studies in massive bleeding in connection with trauma. Case reports and preliminary reports from clinical studies have shown positive results both in these conditions and in other forms of serious bleeding.

The hemostatic effect of NovoSeven is diminished in pronounced acidosis (pH below 7.2), low fibrinogen (below 1.0 g/L) and possibly also when platelet count is below $50–100 \times 10^9$/L.

The doses and dosage schedule for NovoSeven in connection with massive bleeding or other serious bleedings in adults have varied around 0.1 mg/kg bodyweight as IV bolus during 2–3 minutes. NovoSeven can be combined with tranexamic acid.

Concentrates of other coagulation factors

In occasional cases, addition of FVIII, FXIII and VWF (Haemate) can be required when levels of the factor in question have been found to be low.

Cryoprecipitates

In many countries cryoprecipitates are used to compensate for coagulation defects. They contain high amounts of fibrinogen, FXIII, FVIII and VWF.

For factor concentrates and dosages, see Chapter 4.

Tranexamic acid

Tranexamic acid is a fibrinolysis inhibitor, inhibiting the activation of plasminogen to plasmin. It is excreted via the kidneys. The half-life in normal kidney function is about 80 minutes.

Dosage is 10–20 mg/kg bodyweight 3–4 times/24 h IV in normal kidney function; higher doses have been used in cardiac surgery. There is uncertainty about the optimal dosage.

Note that tranexamic acid can cause clot formation in kidneys, urethra and bladder during ongoing bleeding in the urinary tract.

Tranexamic acid can also be used as a local hemostatic drug, e.g. in bleeding from the mouth, nose, rectum or a wound. For preparation and dosage, see Chapter 4.

Desmopressin

Desmopressin has no significant hemostatic effect in connection with trauma and massive bleeding but can be useful if there is a simultaneous platelet function defect or in certain forms of VWD. Desmopressin is often combined with tranexamic acid.

For dosage and special considerations for treatment, see Chapter 4.

Local hemostatic drugs

Local hemostatic drugs can be helpful in serious bleeding. They are available in various forms as biologic tissue glues type Tisseel Duo Quick and Floseal. Tranexamic acid can also be used as a local hemostatic drug.

Complicating factors

Kidney failure

Impaired kidney function often causes a prolonged bleeding time, partly due to a low hematocrit but also to platelet and endothelial dysfunction. This can partly explain an increased sensitivity to platelet-inhibiting drugs and bleeding tendency from small vessels and capillaries. Paradoxically, there is an increased risk of thromboses forming in larger vessels due to a combination of hypercoagulation and fibrinolytic dysfunction.

In bleeding, desmopressin may have a positive effect. See Chapter 4.

Liver failure

As liver failure progresses, PT(INR) rises as a result of reduced synthesis of coagulation factors. Impaired liver function can also lead to increased fibrinolytic activity in plasma and thus to a lower fibrinogen level and high levels of fibrin D-dimers. Thrombocytopenia is often present due to portal hypertension and an unspecific platelet dysfunction.

In serious bleeding with co-existent liver failure, it may be relevant to treat with vitamin K, plasma, prothrombin-complex concentrate, fibrinolysis inhibitors and platelet transfusion.

Reduced vitamin K resorbtion
In certain situations, vitamin K deficiency can contribute to elevation of PT(INR), due to defective intestinal resorption.

Malignancies
Blood malignancies, such as promyelocytic leukemia, as well as disseminated cancer and primarily prostate cancer, can initiate markedly increased fibrinolytic activity, with a low fibrinogen concentration and increasing levels of fibrin D-dimers. Besides affecting fibrin, the fibrinolytic activity degrades coagulation factors V, VIII, XIII and the big multimeric forms of VWF; furthermore, it blocks the membrane receptors on the platelet surface, making them, reversibly, less, functional.

In serious bleeding, treatment with fibrinolysis-inhibiting drugs must come first and, when needed, substitute with plasma, fibrinogen, platelets and VWF concentrate.

Ongoing treatment with platelet-inhibiting and antithrombotic drugs

The combination of platelet inhibitory and antithrombotic drugs may result in an additive and potent inhibition of hemostasis, with impaired platelet function, inhibition of coagulation factors and increased fibrinolysis. See Chapters 7, 8, 9 and 10.

Investigation of increased bleeding tendency

CHAPTER 6

Nils Egberg[1] and Margareta Holmström[2]

[1] Department of Molecular Medicine and Surgery, Coagulation Research, Karolinska Institutet; Clinical Chemistry, Karolinska University Hospital, Solna, Stockholm, Sweden

[2] Department of Medicine, Coagulation Unit, Karolinska Institutet, Hematology Centre, Karolinska University Hospital, Solna, Sweden

Introduction

When investigating an increased bleeding tendency, a detailed history is important. With regard to sampling, a number of screening analyses are of primary interest.

If the patient presents with only small, shallow bruises, has no heredity and the screening analyses are normal, there is generally no need for further investigations. But if the patient has a manifest history of bleeding and/or heredity, a coagulation specialist should be consulted even if the screening analyses appear to be normal.

Diagnosis

The keystone of the diagnosis is the history of bleeding (Box 6.1), which is often more instructive than many laboratory analyses. The history is informative preoperatively and in connection with an investigation of hemostatic defects. Further investigation is usually based on the bleeding history and the results of screening analyses.

Evaluating a case history can be difficult and calls for experience to distinguish between what may be normal as opposed to definitely pathologic. Spontaneous muscle or joint bleeding is almost always associated with severe hemophilia or other total coagulation factor deficiencies, sometimes also with severely defective platelet function. If nose bleeds or

Essential Guide to Blood Coagulation. By Jovan P. Antovic and Margareta Blombäck
© Blackwell Publishing, ISBN: 9781405196277

Box 6.1 Suggested questions for bleeding history (yes/no)

Do you bruise easily?

Do you often have nose bleeds?

Do you bleed abnormally from a cut or other wound?

Do your gums often bleed?

Have you had any muscle bleedings?
   If yes, what was the cause?

Have you had any joint bleedings?
   If yes, what was the cause?

Have you had a tooth extracted?
   If yes, did you bleed for more than 5 hours afterwards?

Have you undergone any surgery?
   If yes, what for?

Have you bled abnormally after surgery?

Have you been given blood or plasma for bleeding from surgery?

Do you have plentiful menstrual bleeding (menorrhagia)?

Have you had a delivery?

Have you had abnormal bleeding after a delivery/abortion?
   If so, did you receive transfusion of blood or plasma?

Which drugs do you use (including contraceptives)?

Do you suffer from any liver, kidney or blood disease?

Heredity – have any of your relatives had problems with bleeding after surgery, delivery or tooth extraction?

---

bleeding after tooth extraction or menorrhagia have required hospital treatment, they are also more likely to indicate a hemostatic defect. Frequent bleedings, perhaps of various origins, also indicate a hemostatic defect. If a close relative is known to have a verified specific defect, measurement of the factor in question is usually mandated.

Laboratory tests
Recommended screening analyses include platelet count, PT(INR), APT time, fibrinogen and bleeding time. See also Chapter 3.

Reasons for pathologic screening analyses and further actions

- If bleeding time is prolonged in a patient with no history of bleeding, repeat the measurement with skilled personnel and if this confirms the first measurement, contact a coagulation expert. Note that bleeding time lengthens during pregnancy (normally not above the upper reference limit) and is prolonged in connection with decreasing extravascular fluid.
- Drug effects (ASA, clopidogrel, NSAID, antiepileptics and certain antidepressive drugs). For patients with a bleeding time of more than 900 s, who do not respond to desmopressin (Octostim®) (see also Chapter 4), request an investigation with certain special platelet tests (a referral to a coagulation unit is advisable).
- Thrombocytopenia (platelet count below $80 \times 10^9/L$). For causes, see below. The number of platelets is crucial for adequate primary hemostasis. Levels above $50 \times 10^9/L$ are usually sufficient but bleeding time can be prolonged even at $80 \times 10^9/L$.

To investigate thrombocytopenia when a coagulation disorder is not likely, contact a hematologist. In this context, hemostatic disorders include the following.

- *Von Willebrand's disease (VWD)*. However, bleeding time may be normal in a mild form of VWD. Analyze VWF (VWF functional =VWF:RCo and VWF antigen) and FVIII and calculate the ratios FVIII/VWF:Ag and VWF:Ag/VWF:RCo.
- *Acquired platelet function defects* due to liver damage, kidney damage, autoimmune disease such as SLE, platelet inhibitory drugs, increased fibrinolysis.
- *Hereditary platelet function disorders*, e.g. Glanzmann's thrombasthenia and Bernard–Soulier syndrome.
- *Disseminated intravascular coagulation (DIC)*. Platelets are consumed as a result of extensive activation of coagulation. Peripheral bleedings (e.g. ecchymoses and bleeding in the gums) already indicate if the bleeding time is prolonged and therefore bleeding time measurements are not necessary.
- Bleeding time may be prolonged in FV and FXI deficiency.

Causes of thrombocytopenia

So-called pseudo-thrombocytopenia is often caused by platelet aggregation in EDTA tubes. Check platelet count in citrate tubes or heparin tubes for comparison.

The following are usually handled by a hematologist.

Hereditary thrombocytopenias
- Isolated (autosomal dominant)
- Combined with qualitative defect (e.g. Bernard–Soulier (see above), May–Hegglin, Wiscott–Aldrich)
- Combined with other defects (e.g. VWD type 2B, Fanconi syndrome)
- Thrombocytopenia with absent radius (TAR)

Acquired thrombocytopenias
Increased peripheral destruction
- Idiopathic thrombocytopenic purpura (ITP)
- Thrombotic thrombocytopenic purpura (TTP) and hemolytic uremic syndrome (HUS). See Chapter Emergency Conditions
- Drugs (i.e. heparin) See Chapter 14 (HIT)

Reduced production
- Aplastic anemia
- Malignant blood diseases
- Metastases to bone marrow from tumors, e.g. breast cancer
- Drugs
- Megaloblastic anemia, B12 or folate deficiency
- Alcohol damage to bone marrow

Abnormal distribution
- Sequestering in an enlarged spleen

Causes of prolonged activated partial thromboplastin time

Check that the sampling was not done with a heparinized needle and whether or that the patient is treated with low molecular or standard heparin (LMH/UFH).

Possible causes
- UFH treatment (LMH can also cause some prolongation of APT time)
- AVK treatment
- Hemophilia A/B; often also in more severe forms of VWD
- FXI deficiency
- FXII deficiency (APT time often greatly prolonged). By itself, this deficiency does not lead to an increased bleeding tendency
- Deficiency of any of the coagulation factors II (prothrombin) and FX can also cause a prolonged APT time; such deficiencies are usually demonstrated better in a PT(INR) analysis

- Circulating anticoagulants (antibodies against a coagulation factor)
- Lupus anticoagulant/phospholipid antibodies
- Severe liver insufficiency

Activated partial thromboplastin time is *not* prolonged in deficiency of FVII or FXIII.

Note that a normal APT time does not rule out mild coagulation disorders, such as mild hemophilia A or B or VWD. So if a disorder is still suspected clinically even though APT time is normal, a specific coagulation factor investigation should be performed.

Causes of elevated PT(INR)

- Liver damage with defective synthesis of coagulation factors.
- AVK treatment: Waran® (warfarin), Sintroma® (acenocoumarol), Marcoumar® (phenprocoumon) or treatment with thrombin inhibitors.
- Vitamin K deficiency (resorption disorder), IV nutrition for more than 5 days, long-term antibiotic treatment.
- Hereditary coagulation defect (FVII, FX, FII = prothrombin).
- Amyloidosis (can cause acquired FX deficiency).
- Antibodies against any of above-mentioned factors or against tissue factor. A pronounced lupus anticoagulant sometimes elevates PT(INR).
- Newborns and healthy children up to 2 years of age have elevated PT(INR) values.
- Seriously ill and prematurely born children have abnormally high PT(INR) values compared with healthy newborns.
- Disseminated intravascular coagulation.

Investigation of bleeding tendency – practical aspects

Elective investigation in nonacute bleeding tendency

Referrals for consultation can be sent to coagulation specialists in the local or referral hospital. The referral must include the bleeding history and results of screening tests.

Preoperative investigation

A preoperative investigation is required in order to avoid unnecessary bleeding complications. Take a bleeding history and, if this is positive, screening samples. In urgent cases, contact the on-call coagulation doctor. If the patient has thrombocytopenia only, contact a hematologist.

Acute investigation in postoperative or post-traumatic bleeding

For patients with a known bleeding disease, always *immediately* contact the on-call coagulation doctor at the referral hospital or the patient's regular center for proposals concerning sampling and treatment. See Chapter 4.

For other patients, first determine platelet count, APT time, PT(INR) and fibrinogen.

Thromboembolic disorders

PART 3

Venous thrombosis and pulmonary embolism

CHAPTER 7

Anders Carlsson

Department of Medicine, Capio St Göran Hospital, Stockholm, Sweden

Introduction

In a US study the average yearly incidence of first lifetime venous thromboembolism among white people between 1966 and 1990 was 117 per 100,000 people. Similar results have been found in the EU with an incidence of 183 per 100,000 people. The incidence increases exponentially with age for men and women, and for both deep venous thrombosis (DVT) and pulmonary embolism (PE). Of the patients with venous thrombosis, 20–30% have either had a surgical event in the past month or have recently had a leg injury requiring a cast or other immobilization. A known malignancy is present in at least 10–15%.

With advancing age, other thrombogenic factors play an increasingly important role (venous status, obesity, reduced mobility, pregnancy, malignancies, autoimmune conditions, estrogen treatment, oral contraceptives, postmenopausal hormone replacement and prostate cancer treatment). Several hereditary coagulation disorders are associated with an increased risk of thrombosis. More needs to be known about the causes of hereditary venous thromboembolism; identified defects account for only about 50% of cases.

Incidence of thrombosis in different clinical materials

The figures mentioned in Table 7.1 refer to the frequency of spontaneous DVT when thrombosis prophylaxis is not given. The ratio of symptomatic to asymptomatic DVT is approximately 1:10. Prophylaxis is nowadays an established practice in connection with surgery.

Essential Guide to Blood Coagulation. By Jovan P. Antovic and Margareta Blombäck
© Blackwell Publishing, ISBN: 9781405196277

Table 7.1 Average frequency of asymptomatic and symptomatic DVT diagnosed in well-controlled studies of more than 10,000 patients

	Percentage
Medicine	
Stroke	20–50 (in the paretic leg)
Acute myocardial infarction	5–30
Surgery	
Elective hip surgery	59
Hip fracture surgery	53
General surgery	29
Neurosurgery	29
Gynecologic surgery	19
Prostate surgery, transurethral	11
Average frequency of lethal PE	
All kinds of surgery	0.8
Hip fracture surgery	7.1
Elective hip surgery	2.4
Trauma (different types)	1.0
Stroke	1–2
Infectious disorders	0.7
Acute internal medicine	0.4

There is no up-to-date information about the incidence of DVT and severe PE in patients with acute myocardial infarction.

Venous thrombosis

Diagnosis
Clinical suspicion

Risk factors for DVT are a previous DVT, recent surgery, trauma, recent immobilization, pregnancy, oral contraceptives of combination types, post-menopausal hormone replacement or estrogen treatment in prostate cancer, infection or malignancy (Table 7.2). DVT can also be due to hereditary defects.

The cardinal symptoms are swelling, burden pain and sometimes, when resting, pain in the thrombotic leg, where an enlarged vein structure and palpation soreness are often observed, sometimes also inflamed superficial veins (thrombophlebitis). Slight fever is a common sign. The more proximal the DVT, the greater is the risk of PE. More than half of all cases of proximal DVT have PE with or without symptoms. Corresponding symptoms

Table 7.2 Medical history/clinical findings in DVT

	Points
Cancer treatment during the past 6 months	+1
Lower leg paralysis or plastering	+1
Recent immobilization for more than 3 days or major surgery within the past 12 weeks	+1
Local tenderness over the deep venous system	+1
Swelling of the entire leg	+1
Calf >3 cm thicker than the other calf, measured 10 cm below tuberositas tibiae	+1
Pitting edema only in the leg with symptoms	+1
Enlarged superficial collateral veins	+1
Earlier documented venous thrombosis	+1
Other diagnosis at least as plausible as DVT	−2

Total points: <1 p = low probability; 1–2 p = medium probability; >2 p = high probability of DVT.

are sometimes seen in an arm affected by a venous thrombosis, and such venous thrombosis may also cause PE.

Differential diagnoses

Erysipelas, *Borrelia* infection, ruptured Baker cyst, ruptured Achilles tendon, bruised or ruptured muscle, venous insufficiency, cardiac failure, hypoalbuminemia, etc. An instrument for standardizing anamnestic statements and estimating the probability of a diagnosis of DVT is provided by the Wells' score.

Tools for confirming or excluding clinical suspicion of venous thrombosis

Ultrasound diagnostics (ultrasound with Doppler, mapping the flow)

A noninvasive method, shown in meta-analyses to have a sensitivity of 96% and a specificity of 93%, compared with phlebography in DVT with symptoms. The sensitivity is considerably lower (less than 60%) in asymptomatic DVT. For DVT in the veins of the lower leg, the sensitivity is about 89%.

Limitations: the accuracy of the method is dependent on the skill of the examiner. The method is more time-consuming for examining calf veins.

Phlebography (venography)

This used to be the most common method, and it is still used as a reference in comparative studies of different methods for diagnosing DVT (in both upper and lower extremities). Phlebography is used when a diagnosis with ultrasound is uncertain and there is a strong clinical suspicion. If the result disagrees with the clinical picture, it is important to bear in mind that a distal or a nonocclusive, more proximal DVT may have been overlooked. A *direct finding* is a picture of a thrombosis surrounded by contrast. An *indirect finding* is failure of contrast to fill the veins; however, this may be due to causes other than a thrombosis.

Limitations: phlebography requires intravenous injection of contrast, which should be avoided in kidney failure and/or treatment with certain drugs (metformin). Distinguishing a new thrombosis from older clots in phlebographic images can be difficult. The method cannot always exclude DVT proximal of the inguinal ligament because of intestinal content, obesity, degree of contrast filling, etc.

Computed tomography (CT)

Computed tomography can demonstrate a thrombosis in sizeable veins, e.g. vena cava superior and inferior, vv iliaca, vv axillaris, vv subclavia and thromboses in splanchnic vessels.

Limitations: requires intravenous contrast injection, which should be avoided in kidney failure and/or treatment with certain drugs (metformin). Computed tomography is often suboptimal for diagnosis of venous thrombosis in cerebral sinus, since the image is symmetric and difficult to evaluate.

Magnetic resonance angiography

Magnetic resonance (MR) angiography can visualize a thrombosis in all large veins. It may be the method of choice for diagnosing DVT during pregnancy, if ultrasound examination fails to confirm the diagnosis. MR is a priority method for confirming clots in cerebral vein sinus. One advantage is that it provides some information even without injection of contrast or at least requires less contrast than phlebography.

Limitations: MR is not always available and is not yet established for DVT examinations. The usual contraindications for magnetic resonance technique apply.

Analysis of D-dimer

There are various methods for analyzing fibrin D-dimer, with a wide range of sensitivity and specificity. Plasma levels of fibrin D-dimer do not differ between women and men. It is primarily a *negative* predictor, i.e. an unelevated level, together with other clinical signs, may be a basis for excluding thrombosis. *Limitations:* the result is difficult to evaluate. Not enough is known about D-dimers in recurrent thrombosis. In hospitalized elderly people and patients with multiple illnesses the level is often increased without a confirmed venous thrombosis. Pregnancy often causes a spontaneous increase in D-dimer levels. Bleeding and inflammation may cause an increase. See Chapter 3.

Superficial thrombophlebitis

Inflammatory conditions may be found in superficial veins because of endothelial damage in connection with local trauma, peripheral vein needle, infection, drugs that irritate vessels, etc. Varicose veins seem to increase the risk of phlebitis. Venous thrombophlebitis is a secondary phenomenon in Behçet's syndrome, Buerger's disease (thromboangiitis obliterans) and malignancy. Such a thrombophlebitis can occur together with DVT, and therefore an exact physical status is important.

Phlebitis in v saphena magna or parva, emptying directly into the deep venous system, is a possible source of PE. With the clinical sign of this superficial phlebitis, it may also be necessary to exclude DVT as well as PE in the patient, because the treatment will change.

Investigation of the coagulation system is usually not indicated, but in exceptional cases, especially in younger patients, it may be advisable to analyze antithrombin, protein C, protein S and mutation FV Leiden.

Pulmonary embolism

Clinical suspicion

Given a clinical suspicion of PE, *prompt and adequate action* is critical. Risk factors for PE are previous venous thromboembolism, recent surgery, trauma, recent immobilization, oral contraceptives, estrogen treatment, hormone replacement treatment (HRT), either postmenopausal or against prostate cancer, pregnancy, infection and malignancy. Some patients have a known heredity for DVT/PE (venous thrombophilia).

The cardinal symptom of PE is impaired physical capacity with symptoms of breathlessness (dyspnea). The symptoms can appear relatively suddenly but can also fluctuate and worsen over time (usually within a week). Various types of arrhythmia, dizziness, chest pain and retrosternal nonprecise discomfort may occur. Ten percent or less of the patients have complaints such as pleuritic pain or hemoptysis. Dizziness and fainting can sometimes be the first symptoms. A slightly elevated body temperature is common and some patients show increased heart rate and/or fast breathing. The symptoms can often be related to lung function, i.e. in patients suffering from pulmonary emphysema, symptoms become dramatic more quickly than in healthy, often young patients with no pulmonary disorder.

Among patients with symptomatic PE, phlebography or ultrasound examination confirms an asymptomatic DVT in the legs in 40–60%. These findings support a clinical suspicion of PE, which must be considered in the choice of therapy, e.g. thrombolysis. Attempts have also been made to create a system for scoring the diagnostic probability of PE. The example in Table 7.3 is taken from a report by the Swedish Council on Technology Assessment in Health Care (SBU).

Tools for confirming or excluding clinical suspicion of PE
Pulmonary X-ray
The X-ray image is a means of revealing cardiac factors (heart failure, etc.) that would explain the symptoms. It can also provide information about other differential diagnoses (pneumothorax, tumor, emphysema, etc.) and can be a guide in the evaluation of a perfusion scintigram, especially if it shows infiltration and/or emphysema.

Table 7.3 Medical history/clinical findings in PE

	Points
Age 60–75 years	+1
Age above 79 years	+2
Recurrence of earlier embolism	+2
Surgery in the past 12 weeks	+3
Heart rate at rest above 100/min	+1
pCO_2 less than 4.8 kPa	+2
Pulmonary X-ray	
Atelectasis	+1
Unilateral elevation of diaphragm	+1
PaO_2 below 6.5 (kPa)	+4
6.5–7.99	+3
8.0–9.49	+2
9.5–11.0	+1

Total points: <5 p = low probability; 5–8 p = medium probability; >8 p = high probability of PE.

Pulmonary scintigraphy

A complete pulmonary scintigraphic examination includes investigation of both perfusion of the lung with perfusion scintigraphy and ventilation of the lung with ventilation scintigraphy. The combination of defective perfusion and normal ventilation is a sign *mismatch*, which is a classic criterion of PE.

The results of the perfusion scintigram can be divided into three clinical categories.

* *Normal perfusion* excludes PE (except in rare cases with an isolated and not totally occlusive thrombosis/embolus in a main pulmonary vessel).
* *Inconclusive perfusion image*, requiring further complementary examination of the defect image. Provided a contraindication for contrast X-ray is not present, it may be cost-effective to avoid ventilation scintigraphy in favor of the recommended "CT lung" with spiral technique (see below).
* *Clinically conclusive perfusion image*. In most cases this requires simultaneous access to a ventilation scintigram (alternatively, CT lung examination) and a pulmonary X-ray.

Pulmonary scintigraphy has been superseded by CT with spiral technique. However, in cases where contrast injection would be inappropriate, ventilation scintigraphy can be a necessary adjunct to perfusion scintigraphy, provided the scintigraphic image can be evaluated by a professional.

Limitations: scintigraphy (perfusion and ventilation) is usually not available outside ordinary working hours and, compared to CT, it is expensive (gamma-camera, staff, isotope, etc.). The evaluation calls for a high level of skill and experience, and even then the interobserver variation is considerable.

CT with spiral technique (spiral CT)

Lung CT is not yet accepted for excluding PE at a subsegmental level of pulmonary vessels. However, several studies have shown that lung CT is capable of excluding acute PE that would demand treatment, and no high frequency of recurrence has been observed during 3 months' follow-up. Moreover, the latest machines provide significantly better image resolution. A great advantage of this method is the lower interobserver variability, especially compared with scintigraphy.

Limitations: the method requires intravenous contrast injection, which should be avoided in renal failure and/or in treatment with certain drugs (metformin). The method is still not sensitive enough to exclude suspected chronic PE.

Pulmonary angiography

This "gold standard" method is expensive and is being superseded by spiral CT for PE diagnosis. It should be used for clinically suspected PE, when there is a pathologic perfusion scintigram and/or contraindication for adequate anticoagulation treatment. Pulmonary angiography is the first choice for diagnosing chronic PE in which a perfusion scintigram is almost always pathologic. Pulmonary angiography provides a direct measure of the pressure in the right ventricle and the pulmonary artery, which is an advantage.

Limitations: pulmonary angiography requires intravenous contrast injection, which should be avoided in patients with renal failure and/or treatment with certain drugs (metformin). Angiography laboratories are not available in every hospital. The examination requires a specialized team with high competence in evaluating images.

Magnetic resonance angiography
This method has not yet been fully evaluated for PE diagnosis.

Echocardiography
Echocardiography is a valuable method for evaluating myocardial loading. A skilled examiner can extract information about the dimensions (dilation) of the right ventricle, and indirectly estimate the pressure in the right ventricle and pulmonary artery. Echocardiographic findings are important parameters for judging the need for thrombolysis or, in rare cases, thoracic surgery. The right ventricle burden may have causes other than PE. A right ventricle burden confirmed by echocardiography may be an indication for continued investigation of a possible PE. Note that an unconfirmed right ventricle burden does not rule out a submassive/massive PE.

ECG
No specific ECG changes are present in PE. Arrhythmia, not infrequently atrial fibrillation, and/or a sign of right ventricle burden may lead to suspicion of PE. In combination with a clinical suspicion, these findings warrant further investigation.

Cardiac enzymes
Elevated levels of cardiac enzymes (troponin, creatine kinase, pro-brain natriuretic peptide and brain natriuretic peptide) may sometimes appear as a sign of a cardiac burden in the absence of coronary disease.

Arterial blood gas
For diagnosing PE, both the sensitivity and specificity of blood gas analysis are low. A normal pO_2 is found in about 15% of PE patients and pO_2 is decreased in about 70% of patients without PE.

Drug treatment in deep vein thrombosis and pulmonary embolism

CHAPTER 8

Anders Carlsson

Department of Medicine, Capio St Göran Hospital, Stockholm, Sweden

Treatment of acute deep vein thrombosis and pulmonary embolism

Nonpharmacologic treatment of lower-leg DVT

The patient should not be immobilized unless there are special reasons, such as intense pain, manifest edema, a fracture, etc. In order to avoid late symptoms, such as venous insufficiency and post-thrombotic syndrome, with a risk of developing venous ulcers (especially leg ulcers), the patient should start to use a compression stocking class 0–1 in the acute phase. After 4–6 weeks, when the leg is no longer swollen, it is recommended that the patient try a compression stocking class 2 (in exceptional cases, class 3). For lower-leg DVT, the compression stocking should not cover the knee. The basic recommendation is to wear the stocking in the daytime for at least 12 months. If the DVT is minor and confined to the lower leg without symptoms, the stockings can perhaps be used for a shorter time. Use should be prolonged if symptoms are still present after 12 months or the medical history or physical status indicates signs of venous insufficiency. A compression stocking loses its elasticity and effectiveness over time and should be replaced every 6 months.

In rare cases, compression treatment is difficult or impossible, for instance if the patient has a severe arterial insufficiency with intermittent claudication and possibly pain at rest. However, the treatment is usually tolerable if the popliteal artery can be palpated.

Essential Guide to Blood Coagulation. By Jovan P. Antovic and Margareta Blombäck
© Blackwell Publishing, ISBN: 9781405196277

Blood sampling prior to pharmacologic/surgical treatment

The following analyses should precede anticoagulation treatment.

- *B-Hb and B-EVF.* Low levels can imply suspected bleeding or other disease and should lead to caution concerning anticoagulation treatment. High levels can also indicate polycythemia vera or secondary polycythemia and thus an increased risk of thrombosis and/or bleeding.
- *B-PLT.* Low levels can indicate a hematologic disorder with an increased risk of bleeding and should lead to caution concerning anticoagulation treatment. However, an arbitrary rule is that B-PLT $80 \times 10^9/L$ or above is sufficient to keep primary hemostasis intact. High levels can also indicate a hematologic disorder and an increased level (platelet count significantly above $1000 \times 10^9/L$) can be a risk of thrombosis.
- *P-APT time.* A prolonged APT time can occasionally indicate a specific coagulation factor deficiency but is primarily a marker of phospholipid antibodies/lupus anticoagulant and an increased risk of thrombosis. During treatment with unfractionated heparin (UFH) as well as with low molecular weight heparin (LMH), APT time can be prolonged or slightly prolonged, respectively. Antivitamin K (AVK) medication may somewhat prolong the APT time.
- *PT(INR).* The basic level of PT(INR) can be important for the choice of drugs for treating venous thrombosis and PE. Spontaneously elevated PT(INR) is seen in impaired liver function, alcoholism, vitamin K deficiency, primary or secondary liver malignancy, etc. Spontaneously elevated PT(INR) implies an increased bleeding risk but does not necessarily mean that the patient is protected against venous thrombosis. On occasion, one may see patients with a healthy liver but a hereditary deficiency of coagulation factor VII or X, resulting in spontaneously increased level of PT(INR). Bleeding is usually rare in patients with hereditary deficiency of factor VII and more common in those with deficiency of factor X.
- *S-creatinine.* Several anticoagulation drugs (LMH, pentasaccharides, etc.) are dependent on adequate kidney function. As a marker of kidney failure, S-creatinine may therefore be important to analyze for the dosage of these drugs (clearance below 30 mL/min should lead to restriction and dose reduction of LMH, thrombin inhibitors and pentasaccharides).

Treatment involving surgery

Pharmacologic treatment for DVT aims primarily at eliminating the risk of PE by reducing the likelihood of increasing an existing thrombosis.

- *Surgical thrombectomy* is used in rare cases, e.g. isolated DVT in the iliac veins in pregnant women or, in special cases, thrombectomy in the pulmonary arteries.

- *Vena cava filter.* A temporary or permanent filter in the vena cava can be used in special cases to reduce the risk of PE when conventional medication is wholly or partly ruled out (contraindication of anticoagulants in proximal DVT (less than 1 week old), serious bleeding complications during ongoing anticoagulant treatment of proximal DVT (1 week to 1 month old), and certain cases where PE shows up in spite of adequate treatment).
- *Stenting* involves placing a plastic or metal tubular structure in a vessel with a narrow lumen in order to prevent turbulence and/or stoppage in the blood flow. Stenting is now in the experimental stage for treating thromboses in large veins.

Drug treatment in deep vein thrombosis and pulmonary embolism

Anticoagulation is the standard treatment for preventing progression of DVT/PE, leaving the rest to the body's fibrinolytic system. The drugs in use are UFH, LMH, pentasaccharides, thrombin inhibitors and AVK drugs.

If proximal venous thrombosis or pulmonary embolism is strongly suspected clinically and it is estimated that the diagnosis will not be confirmed for more than 3 hours, the patient should, *without waiting for an objective diagnosis*, be given UFH 80 IU/kg bodyweight IV or LMH SC (dalteparin 5000–7500 IU SC or enoxaparin 40–60 mg SC or tinzaparin 4500–6000 IU SC).

Subcutaneous LMH is currently the method of choice for patients with DVT/PE. Patients with venous thromboses and, nowadays, certain PE patients are treated with LMH in open-care units. One side effect of treatment with LMH is, of course, bleeding. The bleeding risk is increased in patients with reduced renal function. Thrombocytopenia (HIT type 2) is rare in treatment with LMH, but LMH should not be prescribed for patients with a confirmed heparin-induced thrombocytopenia.

Several LMH are registered for treatment and available for SC injection. Dalteparin is provided in a dose of 200 anti-FXa U/kg bodyweight daily and tinzaparin in a dose of 175 anti-FXa U/kg bodyweight daily. For enoxaparin, the dose is 1 mg/kg bodyweight twice daily or 1.5 mg/kg bodyweight daily in uncomplicated cases.

Treatment with LMH as above can be effective and safe without laboratory monitoring. When LMH is used at the same time as the start of AVK treatment, it should accompany the latter for at least 5 days and until PT(INR) reaches a therapeutic level, usually 2.0–3.0.

If renal function is impaired (clearance less than 30 mL/min), LMH may accumulate in the patient. UFH can be an alternative because it is possible to monitor with APT time.

LMH can affect APT time differently, depending on the type of analysis, so APT time cannot be used to monitor treatment with LMH.

If LMH is used despite impaired renal function, the concentration can be checked by analyzing anti-FXa. This should be done 3–4 hours after the injection of LMH and the level of anti-FXa should be in the range 0.5–1.2 U/mL. If anti-FXa is above 1.2 U/mL, the patient has accumulated LMH and the dose should be reduced. A single daily dose of LMH is preferable to twice daily if renal function is impaired. If reduction of the dose is indicated, the dose should be reduced at least 30–50%.

Treatment of deep vein thrombosis in patients with malignancy

There is a known malignancy in 10–15% of patients with venous thrombosis. Monitoring of AVK drugs is liable to be difficult in these patients, due to defective liver function, metastases, etc. Today there is evidence that these patients can be treated with LMH alone. The recommended treatment regimen is a full dose of LMH during the first month, followed by a reduction to 75% of the full dose. Continuous treatment is often recommended in these patients, with a regular check-up at least every 6–12 months.

UFH

When a strong clinical suspicion of acute PE or DVT is present, especially proximal to the knee joint, a bolus IV injection should be provided initially, pending a definite diagnosis. The bolus dose is usually either 80 IU/kg bodyweight or 5000 IU IV. If the diagnosis is confirmed and UFH is chosen, a continuous IV infusion of 400–500 IU/kg bodyweight/day is suggested. APT time should be checked once a day (in extensive DVT/PE or a risk of bleeding, the first control is performed within 12 hours). An APT time within the desired range is the aim; the target range may differ between different laboratories. Heparin treatment should continue for at least 5 days after the beginning of medication with AVK drugs and until PT(INR) has reached the therapeutic level, usually 2.0–3.0.

Treatment of superficial thrombophlebitis

Treatment depends on the location and degree of the phlebitis. NSAID and Hirudoid can both be used in minor phlebitis. For phlebitis in v saphena magna or parva, we recommend treatment with LMH (full dose for at least 5 days, followed by 3 weeks at a 25% lower dose). An alternative treatment for phlebitis in these large veins may occasionally still be surgery. In secondary phlebitis, treatment of the underlying cause is obviously required.

Bleeding complications in treatment with UFH and LMH

Bleeding can occur during treatment with LMH as well as with UFH. Both drugs have a short half-life and for moderate bleeding it is sufficient to withdraw the drug.

Bleeding from the injection site, nose or gums is treated locally as the first option (a compress moistened with tranexamic acid, mouthwash with tranexamic acid injection solution diluted 1 + 1 with water, or mouthwash with tablets of tranexamic acid, dissolved in water). Blood-stilling cotton can be used for nose bleeding.

Unfractionated heparin can be neutralized with protamine, 1 mg of which neutralizes 100–150 IU heparin. A maximum of 50 mg protamine should be given IV. If needed, an additional dose may be given IV to reach a desired APT time. It is important to allow an interval of about 3 hours between the two injections of protamine.

The dose should be chosen so that only half of the circulating amount of heparin is neutralized. *Caution is required because a surplus of this antidote causes platelet aggregation and thereby thrombocytopenia, which can increase the risk of bleeding.*

Low molecular weight heparin affects platelet function less than UFH does. Protamine does not neutralize LMH to the same degree that it does UFH. An overdose also has an effect that may lead to bleeding complications in LMH treatment by inducing thrombocytopenia (see above). Protamine 1 mg is said to neutralize the prolongation of coagulation time caused by 100 U anti-FXa).

Desmopressin might be considered for serious bleeding related to treatment with UFH/LMH (UFH causes platelet inhibition and prolongation of bleeding time). Treatment with UFH/LMH can then be continued if the bleeding stops.

Thrombolytic treatment

Thrombolytic treatment should perhaps be used more frequently in treatment of DVT/PE. A drawback is the difficulty of selecting the appropriate patients for this risky treatment. The treatment is performed either systemically or locally, via radiologic intervention with special catheters. However, *thrombolysis is not recommended as a first treatment option even in PE,* unless the patient is hemodynamically stable American College of Chest Physicians (ACCP) 7-2004. Drugs that are appropriate for thrombolysis are t-PA and streptokinase. In addition, reteplase and tenecteplase can be used, though that is exceptional at present.

An objectively visualized DVT/PE is required in routine thrombolytic treatment of DVT/PE. Blood samples should be drawn prior to the treatment for analyses of fibrinogen, Hb, PLT, PT(INR), APTtime, creatinine and blood group.

Thrombolytic treatment and thus the increased risk of bleeding must be weighed in every case against the value of rapid thrombolysis and the possibility of preventing post-thrombotic disorders in the long run. Take advice from a skilled colleague before initiating the treatment! **Prior to treatment, consider possible actions in the event of bleeding complications.**

Venous thrombosis

Thrombolytic treatment may be considered in patients with a thrombosis that is still fresh (especially thrombosis times under 3–4 days). The treatment may be relevant for thrombosis in large veins and the upper and lower legs, as well as in the cerebral venous sinus. In exceptional cases, thrombolysis can be considered in body vessels (vv cava, portae, hepatica, renales, etc.). Thrombolysis is less likely to be successful in a total as opposed to a partial occlusion. **The treatment is associated with a risk of serious bleeding complications.**

"Local thrombolysis" or surgery can be an option for a thrombosis of short duration. In exceptional cases it may be worth considering the use of a "v cava filter" prior to thrombolysis.

Pulmonary embolism

Thrombolytic treatment may be considered in acute or subacute massive PE. *It is not recommended as a first treatment option if the patient is hemodynamically stable.*

Criteria for defining a patient as hemodynamically unstable when thrombolysis is being considered

Objectively confirmed PE and at least two of the following criteria.

- Hypotension with systolic blood pressure <100 mmHg
- Elevated troponin
- At least two of the "triad of death": dyspnea (SO_2 <95% + dyspnea), syncope, heart rate > systolic blood pressure
- Peripheral SO_2 <95% in patients with previously healthy lungs
- Affected right ventricle confirmed by echocardiogram
- High BNP (>500 pg/mL)

Indications may suggest immediate commencement of thrombolytic treatment in patients with hypotension and shock.

Before starting thrombolytic treatment of PE, an objective diagnosis is desired, as follows.

- Echocardiography to determine whether the right ventricle is affected.
- Spiral CT of thorax with confirmed embolus, or
- Pulmonary angiography with confirmed embolus, or
- Perfusion and ventilation scintigraphy with a "high probability" of acute PE.

Thrombolytic drugs

Recombinant tissue plasminogen activator (rt-PA)

Recombinant plasminogen activator has been tested in a variety of doses and regimens in order to arrive at the optimal dosage.

Treatment with UFH in connection with rt-PA should be stopped $1/2$–1 hour prior to thrombolysis of PE by infusion of rt-PA. The infusion of UFH may be resumed immediately or within 1–2 hours after the completion of rt-PA.

Several studies have shown that in massive PE, short-term treatment with a high dose of rt-PA normalizes hemodynamics much more quickly than treatment with UFH alone. In massive PE and shock, thrombolytic treatment seems to cause less mortality than treatment with UFH/LMH. If the patient does not show clear signs of improvement within 24 hours, one must either consider another reason for the disorder or repeat the thrombolytic treatment.

Bleeding complications in thrombolytic treatment

- Treatment should be stopped.
- The effect on coagulation is corrected by supplying plasma (refrigerated storage is sufficient for a *maximum* of 1 week).
- Tranexamic acid.
- Samples should be drawn for analysis of P-fibrinogen. Low levels (P-fibrinogen below 1 g/L) should be dealt with by adding fibrinogen concentrate.

AVK drugs
Secondary prophylaxis in venous thrombosis and PE

Antivitamin K drugs should be administered together with UFH/LMH or as soon as the diagnosis has been determined. AVK drugs are not used in pregnancy on this indication; see Chapter 12.

Monitoring the treatment can be difficult in patients with alcoholism, drug abuse, malabsorption, severe liver function disorder, malignancy, etc.

The most common AVK drug in the Western world is warfarin. Some patients are sensitive to the color in the pills, indigo carmine (E132). Itching or temporary skin exanthema occurs in rare cases. In these patients, prescribe warfarin without indigo carmine. Alternatives to warfarin include acenocoumarol and phenprocoumon (Table 8.1).

Note that head injury or onset of acute focal neurology in patients on AVK or other anticoagulant treatment *always indicates a suspected intracranial bleeding* and requires a neuroradiologic examination (CT of the brain). Note also that in connection with head trauma, some days may pass before symptoms appear because bleeding may take time to develop.

Intensity of treatment

Traditionally, treatment with AVK drugs commonly aims for PT(INR) in the range 2.0–3.0. There is now evidence in favor of less intense treatment

Table 8.1 AVK drugs

	Tablet dose mg	Half-life (h)	Protein binding %
Warfarin	2.5	35–45	98–99
Warfarin without E132	2.5	35–45	98–99
Acenocoumarol*	1.0	9	98.7
Acenocoumarol*	4.0	9	98.7
Phenprocoumon	3.0	160	99.6

* Also a metabolite has an AVK effect and elimination of the drug is dependent on kidney function.

for some venous thrombosis with a low risk. The range aimed for in low-intensity treatment is PT(INR) 1.5–2.0. There is, however, still no clear evidence that low-intensity treatment in high-risk patients reduces the risk of thrombosis relapse. Neither is it yet certain that the risk of bleeding is reduced to a greater extent than with treatment of an ordinary intensity (PT(INR) 2.0–3.0).

The maintenance dose of warfarin sodium is usually 5–10 mg/day (range 1.25–25 mg/day).

A change from hospital to outpatient care with less frequent monitoring of PT(INR) increases the risk of deviations from the goal range of PT(INR). It is therefore desirable to check PT(INR) within a week after discharge from hospital. If it is then within the therapeutic range, the interval between tests may be lengthened successively, but not to more than 6–8 weeks.

The duration of treatment with AVK drugs is designed to reduce the risk of recurrence. There is no evidence that this treatment reduces mortality. The optimal medication time after DVT/PE has been shown to be longer than was earlier assumed. Most patients are probably helped by 6 months of medication after the first DVT/PE. In patients with distal thrombosis and an eliminated risk factor (e.g. postsurgical thrombosis), medication time can usually be shortened to 3 months (if a coagulation investigation is indicated, it is advisable to await its result before discontinuing the treatment).

It may be necessary to extend medication time beyond 6 months in the event of remaining risk factors, such as malignancy, a deficiency of any of the coagulation inhibitors antithrombin, protein C or protein S, presence of cardiolipin antibodies or lupus anticoagulant – in particular with

Table 8.2 Mechanisms for interaction with AVK drugs

Reason	PT(INR)
Interactions with drugs	Increases or decreases
Increased vitamin K intake (spinach, broccoli, sauerkraut, etc.)	Decreases
Decreased food intake (vitamin K)	Increases
Parenteral nutrition for a long time	Increases
Decreased absorption	Decreases
Forgotten to take the tablet	Decreases
Hypermetabolism, increased physical activity	Decreases
Infection with fever	Decreases
Immobilization, decreased physical activity	Increases
Liver disorder (illness, addiction)	Increases
Ginko biloba	Increases
Curbicin (may be due to vitamin E)	Increases
Hypericum	Decreases
Kan Jang	Decreases
Strawberries	Decreases

co-existing systemic lupus erythematosus and possibly also if FVIII is elevated (over 2.3 IU/mL). Moreover, presence of the very common FV Leiden mutation (1691G>A), causing APC resistance, or the prothrombin mutation (20210G>A) in heterozygous form, seems to extend the risk of a thrombosis relapse and accordingly indicates a prolonged medication time. Homozygosity for one or a combination of the above-mentioned defects obviously means a greatly increased risk of recurrence. Irrespective of the outcome of the investigation of the coagulation system, clinical circumstances, such as extended venous insufficiency, obesity, immobilization or decreased pulmonary function, can be a relative indication of a prolonged treatment time. Recurrence of thrombosis in the same leg extends the risk of post-thrombotic complications and is thereby also a relative indication of a prolonged anticoagulation.

After a second DVT/PE event, it seems obvious to provide a prolonged secondary prophylaxis, but medication for more than a couple of years is associated with a gradual increase in the risk of serious bleeding. An alternative to consider in this situation is to lower the intensity of treatment to the goal range of PT(INR) 1.5–2.0, for which there is some support concerning DVT prophylaxis. For patients with a very high risk of recurrence, for instance with malignancy or severe thrombophilic defects, there is a lack of evidence at present for lowering the intensity of treatment with AVK drugs.

If a remaining risk makes it desirable to continue to give AVK drugs after a second recurrence, the treatment should be reconsidered yearly. At reconsideration, compliance, contraindications, any incident that has occurred, etc. should be weighed against the benefit of the treatment, and an active decision should be made to continue or interrupt the treatment.

Termination of treatment with AVK drugs

Treatment of DVT/PE patients with AVK drugs can be ended without first reducing the dose. This is evident from a great deal of experience and there is no evidence that abrupt discontinuation of treatment can lead to any form of complication. If the patient is to be treated with platelet inhibitor (ASA), there should be an interval of at least 2–3 days between the last AVK dose and the first ASA dose in order to avoid the risk of bleeding due to drug interaction. Note that there is still no evidence that ASA has a prophylactic effect in venous thrombosis.

NOTE: PLEASE STUDY ALL POSSIBLE INTERACTIONS WHEN YOU PRESCRIBE AN ADDITIONAL DRUG TO A PATIENT BEING TREATED WITH AN AVK DRUG.

High PT(INR) during AVK treatment

Measures to be taken when PT(INR) diverges from goal range without simultaneous bleeding

- *PT(INR) above 6.* Administer liquid vitamin K 1–3 mg PO or IV. Reduce dose of AVK. Check PT(INR) within 2 days (over a weekend, within 3 days). Particular caution as a high bleeding risk.
- *PT(INR) 4–6.* Possibly administer liquid vitamin K 1–3 mg PO or IV. Reduce dose of AVK. Check PT(INR) within 2 days (over a weekend, within 3 days).
- *PT(INR) 3–4.* Adjust AVK dosage. Check PT(INR) soon after.
- *PT(INR) 2–3.* Traditional goal range for PT(INR) in anticoagulation treatment.

Divergence from PT(INR) goal range accompanied by minor bleeding

- *PT(INR) above 4.* Reverse PT(INR) to a therapeutic goal range, e.g. with vitamin K 1–3 mg PO or IV. Reduce dose of AVK. Check PT(INR) the next day.
- *PT(INR) 3–4.* Reverse PT(INR) to a therapeutic goal range, e.g. with vitamin K 1–3 mg PO or IV. Adjust AVK dosage.

- *PT(INR) 2–3.* Traditional goal range for PT(INR). Consider vitamin K 1–3 mg PO and dose adjustment, depending on the type of bleeding.

Serious or major bleeding in patients on AVK drugs
- Immediately consider reversing PT(INR) to below 1.5.
- Prompt reversal may be clinically crucial for the patient.

Reversing PT(INR) in treatment with AVK drugs

High doses of vitamin K create a resistance to AVK drugs, so repeated small doses (1–3 mg) are preferable. (Vitamin K injection liquid should not be administered in drops. Draw up in mg the amount you wish to inject IV; alternatively, remove the needle of the injection syringe and give the drug perorally.) It takes 6–8 hours for the effect of vitamin K to materialize, which in most cases is too slow in an acute situation. The effect lasts about 24 hours after the dose has been given.

Factor concentrates are available, freeze-dried, in ampoules. Dosage is according to weight and current and desired PT(INR). With this drug, the patient receives coagulation factors directly without volume loading and the drug takes effect promptly. The PT(INR) may be checked about 10 minutes after the dosage, to estimate if the amount of factor concentrate given is sufficient or not. The effect diminishes after 6–8 hours, so simultaneous administration of vitamin K may be indicated for acute reversal of PT(INR).

Plasma (not necessarily fresh frozen) is dosed by weight and current and desired PT(INR). A disadvantage is that acute reversal of PT(INR) in elderly patients is liable to result in volume loading, with a risk of cardiac failure. The preparations (blood grouping, basic tests and thawing of plasma) often cause an unacceptably long delay. The effect of plasma diminishes after about 6 hours.

Hemostatic treatment with other drugs (desmopressin) and other factor concentrates, including recombinant FVII, etc.

See Chapters 4 and 5.

Elective adjustment of PT(INR) in preparation for risk situations, e.g. tooth extraction, surgery, etc.

Tooth encroachment (extraction, etc.)

PT(INR) below 2.4 is recommended and can be obtained by reducing the AVK dose in good time (this time differs between different AVK drugs with different half-lives) before the day of the operation. *Check PT(INR) prior to the operation.* Local hemostatics include tranexamic acid tampon and/or mouthwash, suture, etc. Restore the therapeutic level of PT(INR) as soon as there is no contraindication.

Intramuscular injection is contraindicated. For such injections to be safe, PT(INR) must be reduced below 1.5.

Intramuscular vaccinations are contraindicated without reversing PT(INR) in patients on AVK treatment. However, most vaccines can be injected SC; when in doubt about this, consult a vaccination unit.

Local anesthesia
PT(INR) should be below 2.4. Reduce the AVK dose as in dental surgery.

Minor surgery
PT(INR) below 2.0 is recommended. Reduce the AVK dose and monitor PT(INR). When PT(INR) is below 2.0, supplement with LMH (dalteparin 5000 U SC or enoxaparin 40 mg SC or tinzaparin 4000 U SC) × 1. This LMH dose is maintained until AVK treatment is reinstituted postoperatively and PT(INR) has reached the therapeutic level.

Major surgery and surgery with a high bleeding risk
This includes liver biopsy, spinal-epidural anesthesia, lumbar puncture, gastroscopy/choloscopy with biopsy, joint puncture, abdominal, prostate or orthopedic surgery, etc. PT(INR) below 1.5 is recommended. Reduce the AVK dose and monitor PT(INR). When PT(INR) is below 2.0, supplement with LMH as above until PT(INR) has returned to the therapeutic level.

Note that when surgery under spinal-epidural anesthesia is planned, LMH in prophylactic dosage should be administered *at least 10 hours before surgery*, often the evening before surgery.

If PT(INR) needs to be adjusted prior to acute surgery, see the section on reversing PT(INR).

Action to take to avoid the risk of thrombosis

Low levels of PT(INR)
Monitoring therapy as follows in patients treated prophylactically with AVK drugs, e.g. patients with a mechanical cardiac valve prosthesis or during the first 3 postoperative months in patients receiving a biologic cardiac valve prosthesis.

PT(INR) 1.8–2.0	Adjust the dose of the AVK drug	
PT(INR) 1.6–1.7	Weight below 60 kg	Dalteparin 5000 U SC × 1 or Enoxaparin 40 mg SC × 1 or Tinzaparin 4500 U SC × 1
	Weight above 60 kg	Dalteparin 10,000 U SC × 1 or Enoxaparin 80 mg SC × 1 or Tinzaparin 10,000 U SC × 1

Extra dose AVK drug + increased maintenance dose unless the low PT(INR) is due to a missed dose.

PT(INR) 1.3–1.5   Dalteparin 200 U/kg bodyweight SC × 1 or
Enoxaparin 1.5 mg/kg bodyweight SC × 1 or
Tinzaparin 175 U/kg bodyweight SC × 1

Increase the dose of the AVK drug. Continued outpatient treatment with frequent monitoring of PT(INR).

PT(INR) below 1.3   Consider hospitalization for observation. LMH in full dose or UFH infusion. Adjust the dose of AVK to a therapeutic PT(INR)

Intoxication with AVK drugs

Be sure that intoxication is present. This can normally be done by checking PT(INR). Evaluating PT(INR) must be done in relation to the effect of the AVK drug being used. The longer the half-life, the longer it takes for PT(INR) to be affected. At the same time, the duration of the effect increases with the drug's half-life (see above).

If the patient is bleeding, begin treatment without waiting for laboratory results.

- Check if the patient is bleeding.
- Check P-PT(INR), P-APT time and B-Hb.
- Give active charcoal in repeated doses.
- Consider antidote (vitamin K) when the PT(INR) result is known.
- Consider factor concentrate.
- Consult coagulation specialist on call.

Bleeding during treatment with UFH/LMH, thrombin inhibitors and pentasaccharides

UFH

- Stop the treatment, including UFH.
- Check Hb, platelet count, APT time, PT(INR) (if simultaneous AVK treatment).
- Check APT time, for instance every 4 hours.
- Consider injection of protamine 10 mg/mL. Give 50 mg = 5 mL IV during 10 min (50 mg neutralizes about 5000 U of UFH). The dose can be repeated when needed.
- For serious bleeding, plasma (fresh frozen or stored not more than 2 weeks) can be administered and factor concentrate can also be considered.

- When APT time has reached the therapeutic level, and provided the patient does not bleed, UFH can be reinstituted at an adjusted dose if treatment is to be continued.

LMH

Dalteparin, enoxaparin and tinzaparin have no effective antidote. Bleeding can be somewhat reduced with protamine, which can be administered in the same way as for bleeding due to UFH.

Other treatment according to symptoms.

Bleeding during treatment with thrombin inhibitors or with pentasaccharides

These new antithrombotic drugs do not yet have a known antidote. Bleeding requires symptomatic treatment. Consult the coagulation specialist on call.

Primary prophylaxis against deep vein thrombosis and pulmonary embolism

Thrombosis prophylaxis is recommended in surgery for patients over 45 years of age who are to have surgery for more than half an hour.

There are a variety of methods for preventing DVT/PE. Mechanical methods alone are less effective than drug prophylaxis, and the effect of mechanical methods against PE has not been documented. There are indications, in particular cases, that a filter in vena cava inferior can be used as prophylaxis against PE in patients for whom pharmacologic treatment is contraindicated or liable to lead to complications. A cava filter can be applied percutaneously for both temporary and permanent use.

Physical prophylaxis

Exercise treatment and early postoperative mobilization are important for diminishing the postoperative risk of thrombosis. Bedridden patients should be told to flex their feet up and down regularly and to advance to a bed-bicycle, a chair-bicycle and walking exercises as soon as possible. Exercise treatment by itself is not sufficient to prevent thromboembolism.

Thromboses often occur while surgery is in progress, so it is advisable to improve the venous return by elevating the foot of the bed and using graded compression stockings or intermittent mechanical calf muscle compression during surgery.

Drug prophylaxis with a medical diagnosis

Patients with a known bleeding tendency should not be given LMH or UFH as a routine. On the other hand, a known bleeding tendency (e.g. just a prolonged capillary bleeding time, etc.) does not necessarily indicate a decreased risk of DVT as a postoperative complication.

Patients with medical diseases with a moderate or high risk of DVT/LE may be treated with LMH 5000 IU dalteparin or 40 mg enoxaparin once daily.

Drug prophylaxis in surgery

Low molecular weight heparin (half-lives: dalteparin IV 2 hours, SC 4 hours, enoxaparin SC 4 hours, tinzaparin SC 1.5 hours) is the predominant prophylactic method in surgery. Treatment with LMH starts pre- or postoperatively and is given as dalteparin SC in doses of 2500–5000 anti-FXa units/day or as enoxaparin 20–40 mg/day. The higher dose is used in high-risk surgery (orthopedic, cancer surgery, etc.). In order to reduce the risk of bleeding, the higher dosage usually starts 10–12 hours prior to surgery (normally the previous evening), followed by one injection every evening. In general surgery, the treatment is given for 7–10 days, possibly for as long as the patient is immobilized. In high-risk surgery, the postoperative prophylaxis may be prolonged for 3–7 weeks, especially in patients whose risk profile includes malignancy or an earlier venous thrombosis. Long-term prophylaxis (3–4 weeks) should be considered in particularly high-risk patients with a continued postoperative risk (especially after orthopedic surgery).

For surgery under spinal or epidural anesthesia, thrombosis prophylaxis can be started pre- or postoperatively.

- *Preoperative start.* Provided kidney function is normal, we recommend that epidural anesthesia is not performed until at least 10 hours after the end of LMH prophylaxis.
- *Postoperative start.* We recommend that thrombosis prophylaxis is given as soon as surgical hemostasis permits, preferably as soon as 6 hours after surgery.

Sodium danaparoid (half-life 25 hours SC or IV) is an antithrombotic drug that has been registered for prophylaxis against thrombosis in general and in orthopedic surgery. Until more modern antithrombotic drugs became available, danaparoid was an alternative for patients with HIT type 2. However, this drug is sometimes inappropriate due to cross-reaction with UFH and continued formation of antibodies and thrombocytopenia. Danaparoid is mainly excreted via the kidneys. The reversing effect of protamine in danaparoid medication is not clear and is not recommended. Danaparoid does not have a specific antidote.

Thrombin and FXa inhibitors

Argatroban has been used in the USA for a long time for thrombosis prophylaxis in patients with HIT type 2 and is approved for patients at risk for HIT undergoing percutaneous coronary interventions (PCI). See Chapter 14.

Pentasaccharide, Xa inhibitor

Fondaparinux (half-life 17–21 hours) is registered for thrombosis prophylaxis in major orthopedic surgery. The prophylactic treatment starts not less than 6 hours after the surgery. The drug's half-life makes it advisable to wait at least 36 hours between the injection of fondaparinux and manipulation of the catheter to avoid bleeding, even if normal renal function is present. The drug should be used with great caution if kidney function is impaired. Laboratory monitoring is not normally required. The concentration of the drug can be assessed by analyzing anti-FXa. Fondaparinux has been reported to induce formation of antibodies but it is still uncertain if it can cause clinical HIT type 2. The drug does not have a specific antidote.

For HIT see also Chapter 14. For rivaroxaban and dabigatran, see Chapter 9.

Dextran is a plasma expander with flow-enhancing and antihemostatic properties that provides protection against thrombosis and PE. In order to counteract anaphylactic reactions, 20 mL of hapten-inhibiting low molecular dextran should be given first, followed after a few minutes by 500 mL dextran as an IV infusion. An additional 500 mL is given within the first 24 hours and the following day. In hip surgery, 500 mL dextran can be given every second day by infusion. This has to be repeated if more than 48 hours have passed since the latest dose. Caution is required in elderly patients with latent heart failure (cardiac overloading) and in dehydrated patients (risk of kidney damage).

AVK drugs

Antivitamin K drugs have a prophylactic antithrombotic effect in connection with surgery. However, as such treatment is difficult to monitor, it entails a greater risk of bleeding compared to treatment with LMH, UFH or dextran.

Platelet inhibitors

Acetylsalicylic acid and other platelet-inhibiting drugs have been tested as prophylactics in DVT/LE, alone or in various combinations. Their effect has not been established.

New anticoagulants: focus on currently approved oral factor Xa and factor IIa inhibitors

CHAPTER 9

Rickard E. Malmström

Department of Medicine, Clinical Pharmacology Unit, Karolinska Institutet; Karolinska University Hospital, Solna, Stockholm, Sweden

Introduction

Several direct oral inhibitors of factor Xa and factor IIa (thrombin) are currently in clinical development. These agents may have pharmaceutical and pharmacologic advantages compared with low molecular weight heparins and vitamin K antagonists in short- and long-term anticoagulation treatment, respectively. This chapter will focus on the most advanced direct oral inhibitors of factor Xa (rivaroxaban) and factor IIa (dabigatran) and their currently approved indications in the prevention of venous thromboembolism (VTE) in adult patients undergoing elective hip or knee replacement surgery.

Rivaroxaban

Rivaroxaban (Xarelto®, Bayer HealthCare AG) is an oral low molecular weight direct factor Xa (FXa) inhibitor. Rivaroxaban inhibits FXa by binding to its active site. The inhibition is dose dependent and can be measured by prolongation of prothrombin time (PT). Data from phase I studies show that 15 mg of rivaroxaban reduces FXa activity by 35% and increases PT 1.4-fold compared with basal levels. The prolongation of PT is strongly correlated to plasma levels of rivaroxaban (r = 0.935), with little interindividual variability [1]. Thus, the determination of PT seems to be a useful tool for therapeutic monitoring of rivaroxaban treatment, if necessary. The method is, however, not in current routine clinical use.

After oral administration, rivaroxaban is rapidly absorbed, with 80% bio-availability. Maximal plasma concentrations are achieved with 2.5–4 h.

Essential Guide to Blood Coagulation. By Jovan P. Antovic and Margareta Blombäck
© Blackwell Publishing, ISBN: 9781405196277

After multiple dosing, the half-life is 5–9 h in healthy volunteers and 9–13 h in the elderly (average 65 years). Elimination is dependent on the absorption rate; with a 10 mg dose, the half-life has been reported to be 7–11 h [2]. No significant circulating active metabolite has been identified. About a third of an ingested dose of rivaroxaban is renally excreted in an unchanged form. The remaining two-thirds are metabolized in the liver [3]. Elimination is reduced in old age, in cases of decreased renal function and in the presence of strong inhibitors of CYP3A4 (e.g. azole antimycotics such as ketoconazole and protease inhibitors such as ritonavir). In patients with severe renal insufficiency (creatinine clearance <30 mL/min), plasma concentrations of rivaroxaban have been reported to be increased by 64% and PT was prolonged by 144% (p < 0.001) compared with control subjects [4]. Patients with creatinine clearance below 30 mL/min and those with significant liver disease or ongoing medication with strong CYP3A4 inhibitors/inducers were excluded in the phase III studies.

Preclinical data indicate that recombinant activated factor VII (rFVIIa) could potentially be used for partial reversal of the effects of rivaroxaban [5]. In a rat mesenteric model of bleeding, rFVIIa was administered after a high dose of rivaroxaban (2 mg/kg). A dose of rFVIIa at 400 μg/kg reduced the bleeding time by nearly 50% and partially reversed the prolongation of PT and total thrombin activity, without affecting rivaroxaban-dependent FXa inhibition. These preclinical data must, however, be confirmed in clinical trials to establish their clinical relevance.

Clinical efficacy and safety of rivaroxaban

Rivaroxaban at doses of 2.5–30 mg twice daily and 5–40 mg once daily (od) demonstrated a flat dose–response association as regards the effects on venous thromboembolic events in phase II studies [2]. In contrast, the risk of bleeding was clearly dose dependent. At doses of 20 mg per day (od or divided into two daily doses) or more, the risk of major bleeding was 4% and above, whereas at doses of up to 10 mg per day this risk was 0.7–2.3% (without an evident dose–response in the interval of 5–10 mg per day, od or divided into two daily doses). With this background, the 10 mg od dose was chosen for the phase III program.

To summarize the phase III studies [6–8], rivaroxaban (10 mg od PO) demonstrated superior efficacy to enoxaparin (40 mg od SC). The number of subjects included in these studies was enough to show statistically significant superiority of rivaroxaban compared with enoxaparin for the prevention of thromboembolic events, i.e. the commonly used surrogate endpoint of VTE detected by means of routine venography, after elective knee or hip replacement surgery.

The randomized, double-blind, phase III studies RECORD1 (Table 9.1) and RECORD2 included patients scheduled for elective unilateral total

Table 9.1 Rivaroxaban: efficacy and safety in pivotal phase III studies

Study name	RECORD1	RECORD3
Study design	Randomized, double-blind, active control	Randomized, double-blind, active control
Study population and intervention	n = 4541; elective unilateral total hip replacement patients; oral rivaroxaban (10 mg 1×1) starting 6–8 h after surgery compared with enoxaparin (40 mg od SC) starting 12 h before surgery; 35±4 days treatment; follow-up with mandatory bilateral venography	n = 2531; elective unilateral total knee replacement patients; oral rivaroxaban (10 mg 1×1) starting 6–8 h after surgery compared with enoxaparin (40 mg od SC) starting 12 h before surgery; 10–14 days treatment; follow-up with mandatory bilateral venography
Primary efficacy outcome	Total VTE events (symptomatic or venographic DVT and/or nonfatal PE) and all-cause mortality	Total VTE events (symptomatic or venographic DVT and/or nonfatal PE) and all-cause mortality
Secondary efficacy outcomes	Major VTE (proximal DVT and PE) and VTE-related death Symptomatic VTE	Major VTE (proximal DVT and PE) and VTE-related death Symptomatic VTE
Safety outcomes	Bleeding events	Bleeding events
Results	4433 patients in safety analysis 3153 patients in efficacy analysis	2459 patients in safety analysis 1702 patients in efficacy analysis
Primary efficacy outcome	1.1% (R) vs 3.7% (E), $p < 0.001$	9.6% (R) vs 18.9% (E), $p < 0.001$
Secondary efficacy outcomes:		
Major VTE/VTE-related death	0.2% (R) vs 2.0% (E), $p < 0.001$	1.0% (R) vs 2.6% (E), $p = 0.016$
Symptomatic VTE	0.3% (R) vs 0.5% (E), $p = 0.22$	0.7% (R) vs 2.0% (E), $p < 0.005$
Any bleeding	6.0% (R) vs 5.9% (E), $p = 0.94$	4.9% (R) vs 4.8% (E), $p = 0.93$
Major bleeding	0.3% (R) vs 0.1% (E), $p = 0.18$	0.6% (R) vs 0.5% (E), $p = 0.77$
Nonmajor bleeding	5.8% (R) vs 5.8% (E)	4.3% (R) vs 4.4% (E)
Liver enzyme elevation	2.0% vs 2.7%	1.7% vs 1.7%

R, rivaroxaban; E, enoxaparin
ALT, Alanine Aminotransferase > 3 × ULN, Upper Limit of Normal

hip replacement surgery. The primary efficacy outcome was assessed in connection with a composite endpoint of deep vein thrombosis (DVT; either symptomatic or detected by bilateral venography if the patient was asymptomatic), nonfatal pulmonary embolism or death from any cause. The numbers of patients included were 4541 and 2509, respectively, and they were randomized to receive either 10 mg of oral rivaroxaban once daily, beginning after surgery, or 40 mg of enoxaparin subcutaneously once daily, beginning the evening before surgery. In RECORD1, active treatment with either drug was continued for 35 ± 4 days. Events connected to the primary efficacy endpoint occurred in 18 of 1595 patients (1.1%) in the rivaroxaban group and in 58 of 1558 patients (3.7%) in the enoxaparin group. The majority of these events were asymptomatic and detected in (mandatory) venography. In RECORD2, active treatment with rivaroxaban was continued for 35 ± 4 days, while treatment with enoxaparin was given for 10–14 days only. The primary efficacy endpoint was reached in 2.0% and 5.1% of the patients in the two treatment groups, respectively. In both studies, the difference was statistically significant.

Efficacy and safety in patients scheduled for elective unilateral total knee replacement surgery were studied in RECORD3 (see Table 9.1), which included 2531 patients. The same composite primary efficacy endpoint as in the RECORD1 and 2 studies described above was used. Active treatment with either drug was continued for 10–14 days. The primary efficacy endpoint was reached in 9.6% of patients in the rivaroxaban group and in 18.9% in the enoxaparin group, the difference being statistically significant. The vast majority of these events were asymptomatic and detected in (mandatory) venography.

The number of subjects studied was too small to allow conclusive analysis of less frequent events, e.g. symptomatic VTE and deaths. Symptomatic VTE were, however, analyzed in RECORD3, and fewer events were observed among patients treated with rivaroxaban (0.7% vs 2.6%) compared with enoxaparin (see Table 9.1).

Preliminary results indicate that rivaroxaban also showed superior efficacy compared with the US-approved dosing regimen of enoxaparin in preventing VTE in patients who had undergone total knee replacement surgery in the RECORD4 trial [9]. This trial involved 3148 patients who were assigned to rivaroxaban (10 mg od) starting 6–8 hours post surgery or to enoxaparin (30 mg twice daily SC) 12–24 hours post surgery. Both treatments were continued for 10–14 days. Patients were followed for 40 days, after which time venography of all extremities was performed. The primary endpoint of total VTE events (defined as the composite of all DVT events, nonfatal pulmonary embolism and all-cause mortality) was significantly reduced in the rivaroxaban group (6.9% vs 10.1%, p = 0.012). Although numerically lower in the rivaroxaban group, there were no significant differences in major VTE (1.2% vs 2.0%) and symptomatic VTE (0.7% vs 1.2%). The rates of any bleeding (10.5% vs 9.4%), nonmajor bleeding (10.2% vs 9.2%) and major bleeding (0.7% vs 0.3%) were numerically greater in rivaroxaban-treated patients.

The safety of the doses of rivaroxaban and enoxaparin studied seemed comparable after 10–35 days of treatment (see Table 9.1). Overall, similar rates and profiles of discontinuation of treatment with rivaroxaban and enoxaparin because of adverse events were observed. Hemorrhage (surgical and extrasurgical site hemorrhage) is a risk. The incidence rate of major bleeding was comparable between the two treatments, but the overall bleeding events were numerically slightly higher among patients treated with rivaroxaban in comparison with enoxaparin (see Table 9.1). The potential for an increased risk of bleeding in association with rivaroxaban still exists, especially in vulnerable patients, as discussed above.

The incidence of liver enzyme elevations in connection with 10–35 days of treatment with rivaroxaban has been similar to, or slightly below, that observed with enoxaparin. In the RECORD1 and 3 trials, the incidence of ALT > 3 × ULN was 1.7–2.0% in rivaroxaban-treated patients and 1.7–2.7% in enoxaparin-treated patients. A few subjects had a concomitant bilirubin elevation. It is well known that transient liver enzyme elevations are observed when LMH are used. This may at least partially be explained by the fasting and recommencing feeding procedure before and after surgery. See further discussion on liver enzymes in the section on dabigatran below.

The long-term safety of rivaroxaban is currently not known. In the ODIXa-DVT study [10], there are data on a slightly longer (3-month) period of rivaroxaban treatment in patients with DVT. During the first 3 weeks of treatment in this study, the incidence of liver enzyme elevation (ALT > 3 × ULN) was lower among rivaroxaban-treated patients than in enoxaparin-treated patients (1.9–4.3% vs 21.6%). After 3 weeks, however, there was a nonsignificant trend towards a higher incidence of liver enzyme elevation in the rivaroxaban group (1.9%, 95% confidence interval (CI) 0.8–3.6 vs 0.9%, 95% CI 0.0–4.8). Treatment with rivaroxaban was prematurely discontinued in three patients because of abnormal liver function test results (two patients died, one with fulminant hepatitis B and the other with carcinoma and liver metastases).

Dabigatran

Dabigatran etexilate (Pradaxa®, Boehringer Ingelheim Pharma GmbH) is the orally bio-available prodrug of dabigatran. After oral administration, dabigatran etexilate is rapidly absorbed and converted to dabigatran by esterase-catalyzed hydrolysis in plasma and in the liver. Dabigatran is a potent, competitive and reversible direct inhibitor of thrombin. Peak dabigatran plasma concentrations occur 0.5–2 hours after oral administration. The mean terminal half-life of dabigatran has been reported to be 12–14 hours in healthy volunteers and 14–17 hours in patients undergoing major orthopedic surgery. The half-life was independent of dose. Most (80%) of the drug is excreted unchanged by the kidneys. The average absolute bio-availability of dabigatran is low, at 6.5% [11]. In healthy volunteers and in patients, the interindividual variability of C_{max} and the area under the concentration curve (AUC), expressed as coefficient of variation, was high, approximately 80%, whereas in healthy volunteers intraindividual variability was close to 30% [12].

Exposure to dabigatran (AUC) was approximately 2.7-fold higher in subjects with moderate renal insufficiency (creatinine clearance 30–50 mL/min) and approximately six times higher in subjects with severe renal insufficiency (creatinine clearance 10–30 mL/min) than in those without renal insufficiency. In elderly subjects, the AUC was increased by 40–60% and C_{max} by more than 25% compared with young subjects. Exposure in female patients is about 40–50% higher than in male patients [12].

Dabigatran etexilate and dabigatran are not metabolized by the cytochrome P450 system and have no effects *in vitro* on human cytochrome P450 enzymes. Therefore, no cytochrome P450-related drug interactions are expected with dabigatran. Amiodarone inhibits the transport protein P-glycoprotein and dabigatran etexilate is a substrate for this transport protein. In the presence of amiodarone the AUC and C_{max} of dabigatran have been reported to increase by 60% and 50%, respectively [12].

There are currently no specific coagulation tests adapted for accurate and sensitive evaluation of thrombin inhibition. The effects of dabigatran have been assessed using APT time, PT, expressed as the INR, and thrombin time (TT). Measurement of ecarin clotting time (ECT), a test which is better adapted to thrombin inhibition but not in current practice in clinical laboratories, has also been used. A curvilinear relationship has been shown between dabigatran plasma concentrations and APT time which is why this test may not be suitable for the precise quantification of the anticoagulant effect of dabigatran [13]. The INR assay has been found to lack sensitivity within the clinically relevant dabigatran plasma concentration range and showed high variability, and is not considered a suitable tool [12]. The TT assay exhibited a linear relationship with dabigatran plasma concentrations, with a high level of sensitivity [12]. However, this assay might be too sensitive for clinically relevant dabigatran plasma concentrations and the reagents used for determining TT in different laboratories are not standardized. A standardized and modified TT assay, of suitable sensitivity, could be a useful tool for monitoring dabigatran. The same goes for the ECT assay, which has been shown to be sensitive to dabigatran and which displayed a linear relationship with drug plasma concentrations over the full range of concentrations [13].

In summary, the pharmacokinetic characteristics of dabigatran, i.e. low bio-availability (6.5%) with great interindividual variability, the concentration–effect relationship and the bleeding risks strongly suggest that drug monitoring is needed, especially in subgroups at increased risk (see below).

There is no antidote to dabigatran.

Clinical efficacy and safety of dabigatran

In a phase II, double-blind, dose-finding study, 1973 patients undergoing total hip or knee replacement were randomized to 6–10 days of oral dabigatran etexilate (50 or 150 mg twice daily, 300 mg once daily, 225 mg twice daily), starting 1–4 hours after surgery, or to subcutaneous enoxaparin (40 mg once daily) starting 12 hours prior to surgery [14]. The primary efficacy outcome was assessed in connection with the incidence of VTE (detected by bilateral venography or symptomatic events) during treatment. A total of 1464 (75%) patients were evaluable for the efficacy analysis. Venous thromboembolism occurred in 28.5%, 17.4%, 16.6% and 13.1% of patients assigned to dabigatran etexilate at 50 or 150 mg twice daily, 300 mg once daily or 225 mg twice daily, respectively, and in 24% of patients assigned to enoxaparin. The major bleeding rates associated with all dose regimens but the 50 mg bid regimen were higher than with enoxaparin. Based on these results, together with pharmacokinetic/pharmakodynamic data (e.g. [13]), it was concluded that therapeutic doses should lie between 100 and 300 mg daily.

To summarize, the results of the phase III studies [15,16], dabigatran (150–220 mg od PO) demonstrated similar efficacy and safety to enoxaparin (40 mg od SC). The number of subjects included in these studies was enough to demonstrate statistically significant noninferiority of dabigatran compared with enoxaparin (dose according to European guidelines) for the prevention of thromboembolic events, i.e. the commonly used surrogate endpoint of VTE detected in routine venography, after elective knee or hip replacement surgery (Table 9.2).

The randomized, double-blind, phase III RE-MODEL study (see Table 9.2) included patients scheduled for elective knee replacement surgery. The primary efficacy outcome was assessed in connection with a composite endpoint of total VTE events (symptomatic or venographic DVT and/or symptomatic pulmonary embolism) and all-cause mortality. A total of 2075 patients were included and they were randomized to receive either oral dabigatran etexilate (150 or 220 mg od), starting (with half the dose) 1–4 hours after surgery, compared with enoxaparin (40 mg od SC), starting 12 hours before surgery. Treatment was continued for

Table 9.2 Dabigatran: efficacy and safety in pivotal phase III studies

Study name	RE-MODEL	RE-NOVATE
Study design	Randomized, double-blind, active control	Randomized, double-blind, active control
Study population and intervention	n = 2101; elective unilateral total knee replacement patients; oral dabigatran etexilate (150 or 220 mg od) starting (with half the dose) 1–4 h (average 3.4 h) after surgery compared with enoxaparin (40 mg od SC) starting 12 h before surgery; 6–10 days treatment (average 8 d); follow-up with mandatory bilateral venography	n = 3494; elective unilateral total hip replacement patients; oral dabigatran etexilate (150 or 220 mg od) starting (with half the dose) 1–4 h (average 3.4 h) after surgery compared with enoxaparin (40 mg od SC) starting 12 h before surgery; 28–35 days treatment (average 33); follow-up with mandatory bilateral venography
Primary efficacy outcome	Total VTE events (symptomatic or venographic DVT and/or symptomatic PE) and all-cause mortality	Total VTE events (symptomatic or venographic DVT and/or symptomatic PE) and all-cause mortality
Secondary efficacy outcomes	Major VTE (proximal DVT and PE) and VTE-related death Symptomatic DVT Symptomatic PE	Major VTE (proximal DVT and PE) and VTE-related death Symptomatic DVT Symptomatic PE
Safety outcomes	Bleeding events	Bleeding events
Results	2076 patients in safety analysis 1541 patients in efficacy analysis	3463 patients in safety analysis 2651 patients in efficacy analysis
Primary efficacy outcome	40.5% (D150), 36.4% (D220) vs 37.7% (E), ns	8.6% (D150), 6.0% (D220), 6.7% (E), ns
Secondary efficacy outcomes		
Major VTEs/VTE-related death	3.8% (D150), 2.6% (D220), 3.5% (E)	4.3% (D150), 3.1% (D220), 3.9% (E)
Symptomatic DVT	0.4% (D150), 0.1% (D220), 0.1% (E)	0.8% (D150), 0.5% (D220), 0.1% (E)
Symptomatic PE	0.1% (D150), 0 (D220), 0.1% (E)	0.1% (D150), 0.4% (D220), 0.3% (E)
Major bleeding	1.3% (D150), 1.5% (D220), 1.3% (E)	1.3% (D150), 2.0% (D220), 1.6% (E)
Clinically relevant nonmajor bleeding	6.8% (D150), 5.9% (D220), 5.3% (E)	4.7% (D150), 4.2% (D220), 3.5% (E)
Minor bleeding	8.4% (D150), 8.8% (D220), 9.9% (E)	6.2% (D150), 6.1% (D220), 6.4% (E)
Liver enzyme elevations (ALT > 3 × ULN)	3.7% (D150), 2.8% (D220), 4.0% (E)	3% (D150), 3% (D220), 5% (E)

D, dabigatran; E, enoxaparin; ns, no statistically significant difference.

6–10 days, after which follow-up included mandatory bilateral venography. The primary efficacy endpoint was reached in 41% and 36% of the patients in the two dabigatran groups, respectively, and in 38% of patients in the enoxaparin group. The vast majority of these events were asymptomatic and detected in the mandatory venography. There were no statistically significant differences between the treatment groups (see Table 9.2).

Efficacy and safety in patients scheduled for elective unilateral total hip replacement surgery were studied in the RE-NOVATE trial (see Table 9.2), which included 3494 patients. The same composite primary efficacy endpoint as in the RE-MODEL study described above was used. Active treatment with either drug was continued for 28–35 days. The primary efficacy endpoint was reached in 9% and 6% of patients in the two dabigatran groups and in 7% of patients in the enoxaparin group. The majority of these events were asymptomatic and detected in (mandatory) venography. There were no statistically significant differences between the treatment groups (see Table 9.2).

The number of subjects studied was too small to allow conclusive analysis of less frequent events, e.g. symptomatic VTE and deaths. It can be noted that in the RE-NOVATE trial, a slightly higher incidence of symptomatic DVT was observed among patients treated with dabigatran (0.5–0.8%) than with enoxaparin (0.1%; see Table 9.2).

In the double-blind, randomized RE-MOBILIZE trial [17], dabigatran was compared with the US-approved dosing regimen of enoxaparin. Patients undergoing total knee arthroplasty were randomized to receive oral dabigatran etexilate (220 or 150 mg once daily), or enoxaparin (30 mg bid SC) after surgery. As in the other phase III studies, the first dose of dabigatran etexilate was one half (110 or 75 mg) of subsequent doses. The first dabigatran dose was administered 6–12 hours after completion of surgery. The first subcutaneous injection of enoxaparin was given 12–24 hours after surgery, usually on the morning after the day of surgery. Treatment was continued for a total of 12–15 days, followed by mandatory bilateral venography. Among 1896 patients, dabigatran (220 and 150 mg) showed inferior efficacy versus enoxaparin (VTE rates of 31% (p = 0.02 vs enoxaparin), 34% (p < 0.001 vs enoxaparin) and 25%, respectively). Bleeding rates were similar. Thus, dabigatran showed inferior efficacy compared with the twice-daily US enoxaparin regimen. The discrepancy between these results and those of the other phase III studies may be explained by the delayed dosing of dabigatran and the more intense dosing regimen of enoxaparin.

Overall, the safety of dabigatran and enoxaparin at the doses studied seems to be comparable at 6–35 days of treatment duration (see Table 9.2). Bleeding events are the most relevant safety issue in specific populations. Analyses of bleeding events in specific populations in the actively controlled VTE prevention trials indicated a clear dose–response association as regards dabigatran. Patients older than 75 years and patients with decreased renal function are especially at risk [12].

The incidence of liver enzyme elevations associated with 6–35 days of treatment with dabigatran has been similar to, or slightly below, that observed in connection with enoxaparin (see Table 9.2). As discussed above, it is well known that transient liver enzyme elevations are observed when LMH are used. This may at least partially be explained by the fasting and recommencing feeding procedure before and after surgery. It should be noted, however, that as regards ximelagatran, now withdrawn because of hepatotoxicity issues, the incidence of liver enzyme elevations observed in connection with short-term treatment was within the range usually seen with LMH. Therefore, even reassuring short-term safety data cannot be considered a guarantee of long-term safety. The long-term safety of dabigatran is currently not known.

Ongoing clinical studies and other therapeutic indications

These two new anticoagulants are also being studied in phase III trials concerning the treatment of DVT/PE, stroke prevention in atrial fibrillation and acute coronary syndromes.

Of obvious interest, from both a clinical and a commercial point of view, is stroke prevention in cases of atrial fibrillation. At present, warfarin is very much underused for this indication, which may partly be explained by the fact that the drug is not suitable for some patients because of its narrow therapeutic interval and the need for perfect compliance, especially in periods of complex dosing. New anticoagulants will presumably not be suitable for some patients either – perfect compliance will still be important. In other patients who could otherwise take warfarin, there may be other factors, including concomitant medication, herbal medicines or food variations, causing fluctuating PT(INR) values. In these patients, it might be advantageous to choose a drug with a lesser propensity for variability. The first oral thrombin inhibitor ximelagatran, now withdrawn because of hepatotoxicity issues, was demonstrated not to be inferior to warfarin in well-conducted stroke prevention atrial fibrillation clinical trials [18,19]. These findings could very well be reproduced with suitable dosing of an appropriate new anticoagulant drug.

Possibility of and need for therapeutic monitoring of new anticoagulants

For short-term treatment indications, e.g. the prevention of venous thromboembolism in adult patients undergoing elective hip or knee replacement surgery, there is a need for therapeutic drug monitoring (TDM), especially in patients among whom there is a risk of higher drug exposure increasing the risk of bleeding. Such patients may include the elderly, those with low bodyweight or impaired renal or hepatic function and those with co-medication with possibly interacting drugs. In possible future long-term indications, e.g. stroke prevention in atrial fibrillation, other situations when TDM is warranted will arise. Such situations include drugs added to ongoing anticoagulant treatment and concomitant disease acquired during treatment. Furthermore, a periodical sample to check treatment compliance could sometimes be indicated – such information is provided by PT(INR) testing in connection with warfarin treatment.

Tests for therapeutic monitoring of the new anticoagulants are not in clinical use today. However, for rivaroxaban a clinically adapted and reliable PT assay could be used. For dabigatran, among coagulation tests, it is probably either a clinically adapted and standardized ECT or TT assay that will provide the best information. Alternatively, plasma levels of either drug may be used.

References

1. Kubitza D, Becka M, Wensing G, *et al*. Safety, pharmacodynamics, and pharmacokinetics of single doses of BAY 59-7939, an oral, direct Factor Xa inhibitor. *Clin Pharmacol Ther* 2005;**78**:412–421.
2. European Medicines Agency CHMP assessment report for Xarelto. www.emea.europa.eu/humandocs/PDFs/EPAR/xarelto/H-944-en6.pdf
3. Kubitza D, Becka M, Wensing G, *et al*. Safety, pharmacodynamics, and pharmacokinetics of BAY 59-7939 – an oral, direct Factor Xa inhibitor – after multiple dosing in healthy male subjects. *Eur J Clin Pharmacol* 2005;**61**:873–880.
4. Halabi A, Maatouk H, Klause N *et al*. Effects of renal impairment on the pharmacology of rivaroxaban (BAY 59-7939) – an oral, direct, Factor Xa inhibitor. *ASH Annual Meeting Abstracts* 2006;**108**:913.
5. Tinel H, Huetter J, Perzborn E. Partial reversal of the anticoagulant effect of high-dose rivaroxaban – an oral, direct Factor Xa inhibitor – by recombinant factor VIIa in rats. *Blood* 2006;**108**:915.
6. Eriksson BL, Borris LC, Friedman RJ, *et al*. RECORD1 Study Group. Rivaroxaban versus enoxaparin for thromboprophylaxis after hip arthroplasty. *N Engl J Med* 2008;**358**(26):2765–2775.
7. Kakkar AK, Bredder B, Dahl OE, *et al*. RECORD2 Investigators. Extended duration rivaroxaban versus short-term enoxaparin for the prevention of venous thromboembolism after total hip arthroplasty: a double-blind, randomised controlled trial. *Lancet* 2008;**372**(9632):31–39.
8. Lassen MR, Ageno W, Borris LC, *et al*. RECORD3 Investigators. Rivaroxaban versus enoxaparin for thromboprophylaxis after total knee arthroplasty. *N Engl J Med* 2008;**358**(26):2776–2786.

9. Turpie A, Bauer K, Davidson B, *et al.* Comparison of rivaroxaban – an oral, direct factor Xa inhibitor – and subcutaneous enoxaparin for thromboprophylaxis after total knee replacement (RECORD4: a phase 3 study). European Federation of National Associations of Orthopaedics and Traumatology Annual Meeting, May 29–June 1 2008, Nice, France. Abstract F85.

10. Agnelli G, Gallus A, Goldhaber SZ, *et al.* Treatment of proximal deep-vein thrombosis with the oral direct Factor Xa inhibitor rivaroxaban (BAY 59-7939): the ODIXa-DVT (oral direct factor Xa inhibitor BAY 59-7939 in patients with acute symptomatic deep-vein thrombosis) study. *Circulation* 2007;**116**:180–187.

11. Stangier KJ, Rathgen K, Staehle H, Gansser D, Roth W. The pharmacokinetics, pharmacodynamics and tolerability of dabigatran etexilate, a new oral direct thrombin inhibitor, in healthy male subjects. *Br J Clin Pharmacol* 2007;**64**: 292–303.

12. European Medicines Agency. CHMP Assessment Report For Pradaxa. www.emea.europa.eu/humandocs/PDFs/EPAR/pradaxa/H-829-en6.pdf

13. Liesenfeld KH, Schäfer HG, Trocóniz IF, Tillmann C, Eriksson BI, Stangier J. Effects of the direct thrombin inhibitor dabigatran on ex vivo coagulation time in orthopaedic surgery patients: a population model analysis. *Br J Clin Pharmacol* 2006;**62**(5):527–537.

14. Eriksson BI, Dahl OE, Buller HR, *et al.* A new oral direct thrombin inhibitor, dabigatran etexilate, compared with enoxaparin for prevention of thromboembolic events following total hip or knee replacement: the BISTRO II randomized trial. *J Thromb Haemost* 2005;**3**:103–111.

15. Eriksson BI, Dahl OE, Rosencher N, *et al.* RE-MODEL Study Group. Oral dabigatran etexilate vs subcutaneous enoxaparin for the prevention of venous thromboembolism after total knee replacement: the RE-MODEL randomized trial. *J Thromb Haemost* 2007;**5**(11):2178–2185.

16. Eriksson BI, Dahl OE, Rosencher N, *et al.* RE-NOVATE Study Group. Dabigatran etexilate versus enoxaparin for prevention of venous thromboembolism after total hip replacement: a randomised, double-blind, non-inferiority trial. *Lancet* 2007;**370**(9591):949–956.

17. RE-MOBILIZE Writing Committee. The oral thrombin inhibitor dabigatran etexilate vs the North American enoxaparin regimen for the prevention of venous thromboembolism after knee arthroplasty surgery. *J Arthroplasty* 2009;**24**(1):1–9.

18. Olsson SB, Executive Steering Committee of the SPORTIF III Investigators. Stroke prevention with the oral direct thrombin inhibitor ximelagatran compared with warfarin in patients with non-valvular atrial fibrillation (SPORTIF III): randomised controlled trial. *Lancet* 2003;**362**(9397):1691–1698.

19. Albers GW, Diener HC, Frison L, *et al.* SPORTIF Executive Steering Committee for the SPORTIF V Investigators. Ximelagatran vs warfarin for stroke prevention in patients with nonvalvular atrial fibrillation: a randomized trial. *JAMA* 2005;**293**(6):690–698.

Arterial thromboembolism

CHAPTER 10

Kenneth Pehrsson[1], Håkan Wallen[2], Jesper Swedenborg[3] and Nils Wahlgren[4]

[1]Department of Cardiology, Karolinska Institutet; Karolinska University
Hospital, Solna, Stockholm, Sweden, [2]Department of Clinical Sciences,
Karolinska Institutet; Department of Cardiology, Danderyd Hospital,
Stockholm, Sweden, [3]Department of Molecular Medicine and Surgery,
Karolinska Institutet; Department of Vascular Surgery, Karolinska University
Hospital, Solna, Stockholm, Sweden, [4]Department of Clinical Neuroscience,
Karolinska Institutet; Department of Neurology, Karolinska University
Hospital, Solna, Stockholm, Sweden

Ischemic heart disease

Stable angina pectoris

Prophylaxis against myocardial infarction: acetylsalicylic acid (ASA)
75–160 mg once daily. In case of ASA allergy, use clopidogrel 75 mg
once daily.

Unstable angina pectoris/non-ST elevation myocardial infarction (NSTEMI)

For signs of instability, such as repeated attacks of chest pain, combined
with ECG changes and/or an increase in troponin-T/I, platelet-inhibiting
drugs should be given in the form of ASA 300–500 mg as a loading dose
followed by 75–160 mg once daily in combination with clopidogrel (75 mg
tablets) given as a loading dose of 4–8 tablets (i.e. 300–600 mg) followed
by 75 mg once daily. The dual antiplatelet treatment with ASA and
clopidogrel should continue for at least 3 months (see below) and ASA
alone "for life" or until serious adverse effects occur. In the acute stage,
combine the above-mentioned drugs with LMH (dalteparin SC 120 IU/kg

Essential Guide to Blood Coagulation. By Jovan P. Antovic and Margareta Blombäck
© Blackwell Publishing, ISBN: 9781405196277

bodyweight/12 h or enoxaparin SC 1 mg/kg/12 h), fondaparinux (2.5 mg SC once daily; in the case of renal insufficiency defined as creatinine clearance 20–50 mL/min, 1.5 mg SC once daily) or UFH (full dose IV) for 3–5 days or until PCI/CABG. In patients with severe renal insuffiency (i.e. creatinine clearance below 20 mL/min) give enoxaparin SC 1 mg/kg once daily.

In cases of peristent instability despite treatment given as above, refer the patient to coronary angiography or if coronary angiography cannot be performed immediately, initiate treatment with a short-acting glycoprotein IIb/IIIa receptor (GPIIb/IIIa) antagonist such as tirofiban or eptifibatide until coronary angiography can be performed. Treatment with a GPIIb/IIIa antagonist should always be combined with LMH or UFH.

The GPIIb/IIIa antagonist treatment should begin at least 12 hours prior to coronary angiography/PCI and continue for at least 12 hours after PCI. LMH (dalteparin or enoxaparin) is, however, discontinued as soon as possible after PCI. If treatment with a short-acting GPIIb/IIIa blocker (i.e. tirofiban or eptifibatide) has not been given, then consider using abciximab (an antibody directed against the GPIIb/IIIa receptor and with a long duration of action) in connection with PCI; this treatment is started at the cath lab.

ST-elevation myocardial infarction (STEMI)

An oral bolus dose of 300–500 mg ASA should be given acutely, regardless of the treatment outlined below. A bolus dose of clopidogrel (4–8 tablets of 75 mg, i.e. 300–600 mg) is also recommended, as pretreatment with clopidogrel is beneficial in both thrombolysis and PCI. Direct coronary intervention (primary PCI) is the first choice in the treatment of an acute ST-elevation infarct. If primary PCI is not available, thrombolysis should be given.

Thrombolysis

Prior to thrombolysis, always check that ASA, and preferably also clopidogrel, has been given (in dosages outlined above).

Tenecteplase is given as a weight-adjusted IV bolus dose, followed by LMH (enoxaparin 30 mg IV *and* 1 mg/kg bodyweight (maximum 100 mg) SC). Continue with ASA (75–160 mg × 1) and LMH (enoxaparin 1 mg/kg bodyweight × 2 SC in keeping with the above) for 7 days or until the patient is discharged from hospital. Thereafter ASA (Trombyl 75 mg × 1) only. Beneficial effects of clopidogrel treatment (75 mg daily) in the setting of thrombolytic treatment have been shown for up to 8 days after the reperfusion treatment, and should preferably be given as well.

An alternative to tenecteplase is streptokinase 1.5 million units in 250 mL of physiologic NaCl solution IV for 1 hour. Continue prophylaxis with ASA (Trombyl) 75 mg once daily, "life long" or until serious adverse effects occur, in combination with clopidogrel 75 mg daily for 1 week. Heparin is given only on special indications.

Developments in this field are rapid at present, so treatment principles often have to be adapted to new guidelines.

Percutaneous coronary intervention

ASA and clopidogrel

Regardless of the indication, all patients should be prescribed ASA (Trombyl 75–160 mg × 1) starting a few days prior to PCI. If this has not been prescribed, a bolus dose of ASA 300–500 mg orally should be given on the day of PCI, followed by ASA (Trombyl 75–160 mg × 1) "life long" or until serious adverse effects occur. In addition, clopidogrel should be given as a bolus dose of 600 mg (8 tablets) at least 2 hours prior to PCI. Depending on the procedure (if coronary stenting is performed and depending on what type of stents implanted) clopidogrel should be prescribed at 75 mg once daily for 1–12 months (sometimes even longer).

Primary PCI in STEMI

Acetylsalicylic acid and clopidogrel in bolus doses as indicated above should be given in combination with LMH or UFH. The GPIIb/IIIa receptor antagonist abciximab should also be strongly considered.

Rescue PCI after thrombolysis without reperfusion
After streptokinase

Abciximab should not be given within 24 hours after streptokinase has been given because of an increased risk of bleeding.

After rt-PA

Abciximab can be given soon after rt-PA if there is an indication (instability and indication for rescue PCI).

PCI-related complications

Abciximab is given in the case of intracoronary thrombus formation and/or embolization, acute occlusions and major dissections affecting coronary blood flow, following excessive coronary stenting and following long-term myocardial ischemia, such as severe chest pain and ST changes on ECG.

Stenting

As stated above, ASA (bolus dose of 300–500 mg followed by 75–160 mg daily) in combination with clopidogrel (bolus dose 600 mg followed by 75 mg daily) is mandatory in coronary stenting. The clopidogrel treatment (75 mg once daily) should continue for 1–3 months if the indication was stable angina pectoris. For unstable angina pectoris, NSTEMI and STEMI, the clopidogrel treatment should continue for at least 3 months, often longer. If a drug-eluting stent (DES) has been implanted, clopidogrel should be prescribed for at least 12 months regardless of the indication. If the patient has an increased risk of bleeding, the duration of clopidogrel treatment could be shortened to 6 months. Of note, DES should preferably *not* be implanted in patients with increased risk of bleeding.

Vein grafts

Abciximab may be prescribed according to the interventionist's judgment.

Diabetics

For unstable angina pectoris, NSTEMI and STEMI, see above. For elective PCI, abciximab is given on wide indications if the interventionist considers that the PCI procedure will be more complicated than normal, such as extended general coronary vessel wall changes, several stent implants, lengthy interventional procedure, etc.

Secondary prophylaxis against arterial embolism

For an anterior wall myocardial infarction with a visible left ventricle thrombus and/or substantially reduced left ventricle function, treatment with an oral AVK drug (e.g. warfarin) should be considered for 3 months or until the thrombus is not visible on echocardiographic examinations or magnetic resonance imaging. Of note, data on warfarin following acute myocardial in the absence of coronary stenting are strong, so warfarin could be prescribed long term instead of ASA. This is especially the case in the presence of severely reduced left ventricle function or atrial fibrillation. Can be given as secondary prophylaxis (i.e. for years or more). In selected high-risk patients, warfarin and ASA could be combined but with great caution as the bleeding risk is considerably increased.

In cases of immobilization consider giving LMH (Klexane 40 mg × 1 SC or dalteparin 5000 IU × 1 SC) during a shorter period if the patient is not receiving AVK treatment.

Cardiac arrhythmias (atrial fibrillation)

The occurrence of atrial fibrillation doubles the risk of mortality in the total patient population. The risk is related to the underlying heart disease. The atrial fibrillation itself is probably of minor importance. The treatment should be adjusted to traditional risk factors. Chronic atrial fibrillation is a common form of arrhythmia and its incidence increases with age. The treatment of atrial fibrillation aims at either rhythm control, i.e. an attempt to convert to a sinus rhythm, and antiarrhythmic treatment in order to maintain the sinus rhythm, or frequency control, i.e. acceptance of the fibrillation with an adequate ventricular frequency regulation (about 70–90 beats/min at rest) and adequate antithrombotic treatment. Recent studies have shown that neither morbidity nor mortality differs between rhythm and frequency control. There is a risk of embolization and stroke, with the following relative risks (numbers within parentheses): an earlier stroke or TIA (2.5), diabetes mellitus (1.7), hypertension (1.6), known coronary artery disease (1.5), heart failure (1.4), age over 60 years (1.4 per 10 years).

Planned electroconversion
If the atrial fibrillation has been present for more than 48 hours an oral AVK drug (e.g. warfarin) should be given daily and PT(INR) values should be 2.0–3.0 for more than 3 weeks prior to conversion. The AVK treatment should continue for at least 4–6 weeks after a successful regularization.

Primary stroke prevention
Low risk of stroke (≤5%/year)
- Under 60 years of age, no cardiac disease: ASA 75–320 mg daily.
- Under 60 years of age and with a structural cardiac disease, but in other respects no known risk factors: ASA 75–320 mg daily.
- Over 60 years of age, no risk factors: ASA 75–320 mg daily.
- Over 60 years of age with diabetes or coronary artery disease: AVK (e.g. warfarin), PT(INR) values should be 2.0–3.0; ASA 75 mg × 1 can be added to patients with a low bleeding risk.
- Age ≥75 years, especially women: AVK (e.g. warfarin), PT(INR) values should be 2.0–3.0.
- Regardless of age, ejection fraction (EF) <35%, thyrotoxicosis and hypertension: AVK (e.g. warfarin), aim for PT(INR) 2.0–3.0.
- Rheumatic cardiac disease (mitral stenosis, mitral insufficiency): AVK (e.g. warfarin), PT(INR) values should be 2.5–3.5.
- Mechanical cardiac valve prosthesis: AVK (e.g warfarin), PT(INR) values should be 2.5–3.5.
- Earlier known thromboembolism or persistent atrial thrombus at transesophageal echocardiography (TEE): AVK (e.g. warfarin), PT(INR) values should be 2.5–3.5, consider combining AVK with ASA 75 mg × 1.

Cardiac valve prosthesis

Embolism prophylaxis with AVK (e.g. warfarin) for 3 months in the case of a biologic valve, otherwise "life-long treatment." If embolism occurs in spite of AVK treatment at therapeutic PT(INR) levels, add ASA 75 mg daily or dipyridamole 75 mg × 3 (data on the latter drug are, however, somewhat weak).

Questions about the above-mentioned treatments should be referred to the cardiologist on duty.

Peripheral artery surgery

Prophylaxis against reocclusion in reconstructive vascular surgery or percutaneous transluminal angioplasty (PTA)

ASA (75–160 mg/24 h), starting close in time after surgery. Clopidogrel (75 mg × 1) may possibly be prescribed. Note that clopidogrel causes an increased bleeding tendency and should, if possible, be discontinued before surgery. Treatment with ASA is primarily prophylactic against future consequences of coronary heart disease and secondarily to maintain patency of the arterial reconstruction.

Perioperative treatment

Intraoperatively, UFH 35–70 IU/kg bodyweight IV or LMH 70 IU/kg bodyweight IV. After surgery, ASA as above. In arterial reconstruction with a high risk of occlusion, AVK drugs (warfarin) can be used postoperatively. Dextran is used in connection with surgery but this should be done with caution due to the risk of fluid overload causing heart failure.

Thrombolysis in acute ischemia

In acute leg ischemia, local thrombolysis can be used. This is usually the case in acute thrombosis caused by an arteriosclerotic disease. A catheter with multiple side holes is inserted through an introducer in the groin for local infusion of rt-PA into the thrombosis. A thrombus in the superficial femoral artery can usually be lysed with less than 20 mg rt-PA. The thrombolytic agent is given in repeated doses of 2 mg and can be followed by a slow infusion of 2 mg/h. Fibrinogen levels are checked with the same routines as for other thrombolytic treatments. The thrombolytic treatment is discontinued if the level of fibrinogen falls below 1 g/L. If the thrombolysis is successful, the arterial stenosis that caused the thrombosis is often visualised and can be treated with PTA with or without stent. In order to reduce the risk of bleeding at the point of insertion, the introducer in the groin is left *in situ* until thrombolysis is completed.

Questions concerning the above-mentioned treatments should be put to the vascular surgeon on duty.

Stroke and transient ischemic attack (TIA)

Secondary stroke prevention

Intracranial bleeding must always be excluded with computed tomography of the brain prior to a decision to initiate antithrombotic treatment.

Acetylsalicylic acid 75 mg daily (first day 300–500 mg as a bolus dose) as soon as computed tomography/magnetic resonance imaging has excluded hemorrhage, although 24 hours must pass since administration of rt-PA. Dipyridamole (200 mg × 2; slow release capsule) after first day in combination with ASA. To avoid commonly occurring initial headache, either start with one capsule before sleep for 5 days before or reduce dose temporarily if headache develops. Clopidogrel 75 mg is an alternative if any of these treatments is not tolerated.

Atrial fibrillation and TIA or stroke

Secondary prophylaxis with AVK (warfarin) should be prescribed in the first place, provided there are no contraindications. The PT(INR) range to aim for is 2.0–3.0. Check PT(INR) regularly. Moreover, AVK (warfarin) should be given in TIA or stroke after recent (<3 months) acute myocardial infarction and also be considered in other kinds of cardiac embolism. AVK (warfarin) treatment can begin immediately after TIA and minor myocardial infarction. In more extensive cerebral infarction of cardiac origin, wait for about 10–14 days and begin the treatment after renewed computed tomography to exclude bleeding.

There are no definite guidelines for the duration of secondary prophylactic treatment. Platelet inhibitory treatment is often given for life. AVK treatment continues as long as atrial fibrillation persists or until there is a risk of complications. After an acute myocardial infarction, the treatment may often be discontinued after a few months. Note that AVK (warfarin) and ASA should normally not be given in combination.

Thrombolysis in stroke

Thrombolysis with IV rt-PA (Alteplase) may be relevant when computed tomography has excluded bleeding and extensive current infarction changes. A marker of extensive ischemia in the area of the median cerebral artery is that the infarction change does not exceed one-third of the volume of the middle arterial territory or one-half of the anterior or posterior artery territories.

Treatment should be given at a stroke unit with experience of this kind of treatment. Patients with very severe symptoms (National Institutes of Health Stroke Score of 25 or higher) should not be treated, neither should patients with an earlier brain hemorrhage, head trauma or a serious disease. An exclusion list must be checked prior to a decision about treatment.

Thrombolytic treatment should be performed within 4.5 hours after the event, although the current European license is still not adjusted for new data and restricts treatment to a time interval of 0–3 hours. Treatment may also be considered beyond 4.5 hours if supported by multimodal neuroimaging indicating reduced focal perfusion with limited established infarct. Thrombolysis should not be attempted after 6 hours, except in cases of intra-arterial treatment of basilar artery occlusion. The time of onset must be stated correctly; if this is uncertain, the last time-point without symptoms is an alternative. In selected cases of unsuccessful intravenous thrombolysis, mechanical thrombus extraction may be an alternative, although this is still a technique under evaluation.

The patient must be treated immediately. Delays in transportation between emergency room, X-ray unit and stroke unit must be avoided. The treatment is given as an intravenous infusion with a dose of rt-PA of (Alteplase) 0.9 mg/kg bodyweight for 1 hour. The effect of successful treatment often appears during the infusion or within the subsequent first hour but may also do so successively during the first 24 hours.

The treatment is associated with a risk of bleeding complications, which can be serious. If intracranial bleeding is suspected during the treatment (a sudden change for the worse, with increasing neurologic symptoms, decreased consciousness, headache), discontinue the treatment (accumulating data indicate, however, that bleeding almost exclusively occurs after the treatment has been finished). If the bleeding is superficial, local compression is performed. If necessary, give refrigerated (stored up to 1 week) or fresh-frozen plasma. Treatment to inhibit fibrinolysis, such as tranexamic acid, may be considered. Contact the coagulation doctor on duty.

Secondary prophylaxis with ASA in a low (ASA 75 mg × 1) or medium dose (ASA 150–300 mg daily) may start 24 hours after the end of the treatment. No data are available on the preventive effects of different low doses of ASA. However, lower doses entail smaller risks of gastro-intestinal side effects. A medium dose may be appropriate during the first days in order to obtain an optimal platelet-inhibiting effect without delay. The preventive effect of ASA may be improved by combining it with dipyridamole, but this should be avoided during the first days because not enough is known about the safety aspect in the acute stage of stroke. Combination treatment may be given as a slow-release capsule (200 mg dipyridamole) twice daily, and a total daily dose of 75 mg ASA. Dipyridamole can sometimes cause initial headache, especially in patients with migraine, but this may sometimes be ameliorated by cutting the dose to one capsule daily for a few days and then returning to two capsules daily.

An alternative to ASA and dipyridamole, if the patient does not tolerate these alternatives, is monotherapy with clopidogrel (75 mg × 1).

Cerebral venous thrombosis and dissection of precerebral arteries

Treatment with UFH and simultaneous initiation of AVK treatment is recommended, provided there are no contraindications. Local fibrinolysis may be considered in cerebral venous thrombosis with progressive neurologic symptoms and/or reduced consciousness. Patients with this condition should be managed at comprehensive stroke centers with capacity for neuroradiologic interventions.

Recurrent TIA

Although random studies provide no support for treatment with heparin, it is often used if the symptoms are suspected to be thromboembolic. The treatment should be avoided, in particular in recurrent lacunar TIA because the disorder is not primarily thromboembolic and the safety of anticoagulation treatment has not been confirmed.

Prophylactic treatment against deep venous thrombosis and pulmonary embolism

A pronounced paresis after stroke entails a risk of deep venous thrombosis and pulmonary embolism. Support stockings are used as a rule in immobilized patients. If paresis persists after the first 24 hours, consider preventive treatment with LMH.

For advice concerning treatment, also in intracranial bleeding and laboratory analyses, contact the neurologist on duty.

Investigations of thromboembolic tendency

CHAPTER 11

Margareta Holmström

Department of Medicine, Coagulation Unit, Karolinska Institutet;
Hematology Centre, Karolinska University Hospital, Solna,
Stockholm, Sweden

Introduction

A coagulation investigation concerning biochemical thrombogenic disorders should be considered above all in relatively young patients (arbitrary limit, below 50 years of age) and in all patients with an extensive heredity. The investigation can be done on samples drawn at a coagulation unit or at other laboratories (samples sent to the coagulation laboratory after contact with a coagulation expert).

The coagulation investigation is usually undertaken in a tranquil stage, as a rule several months (more than 3 months) after the acute episode. However, DNA analysis of mutations can be undertaken during the acute phase. The outcome of the investigation may be influenced by acute phase reactants, estrogen medication (oral contraceptives, HRT), AVK drugs, etc. The result may be important for deciding about further treatment and the investigation should therefore be completed before making a final decision about the length and type of treatment. If the result is not normal, it should be assessed by a coagulation expert.

In the first place, a coagulation investigation in DVT/PE concerns the possible presence of APC resistance, FV Leiden (1691G>A) mutation, prothrombin (20210G>A) mutation, deficiencies of antithrombin, protein C or protein S. In certain cases the investigation can be extended to detect rare defects in fibrinogen, thrombomodulin, FVIII, plasminogen, etc. The presence of phospholipid antibodies, such as cardiolipin antibodies, and lupus anticoagulant may also be related to the thrombotic disorder and should be included in the investigation. Modern studies do not

Essential Guide to Blood Coagulation. By Jovan P. Antovic and Margareta Blombäck
© Blackwell Publishing, ISBN: 9781405196277

support analyzing homocysteine in the investigation of coagulation concerning thrombophilia.

In "unexplainable" (idiopathic) DVT/PE, particularly in elderly patients, remember that phospholipid antibodies can occur in malignancy and autoimmune disorders.

Box 11.1 Thrombosis history

- Have you had a thrombosis in the leg/arm?

- Have you had a thrombosis/embolus in the lung (PE)?
  How many times?
  When?

- Reason for the thrombosis
  After surgery, fracture, confinement to bed, pregnancy, contraceptives
  Drugs? Other disease? Unknown?

- What treatment did you receive?

- Do you have, or have you had, varices?

- Has any close relative had venous thromboses, thrombophlebitis, PE?
  Which relatives and which condition?

- What drugs are you using?

Venous thromboembolism

Possible hereditary defect

Determine APC resistance = B(Lkc) mutation Factor V gene (1691G>A), B(Lkc) mutation prothrombin gene (2021G>A), P-antithrombin, P-protein C, P-protein S free (low levels of the three inhibitors), P-FVIII (P-PAI-1) (high levels of the latter two).

It is usually best to order all these analyses simultaneously. A deficiency of the coagulation inhibitors – low levels of antithrombin, protein C or protein S – is often hereditary.

Abnormal fibrinogen, thrombomodulin and plasminogen can also be a cause of DVT/LE.

Investigation prior to oral contraceptives (OC) and prior to postmenopausal HRT

Women who have had DVT/PE or have a heredity for it should be investigated and oral contraceptives (oc) should not be prescribed, according to gynecologists. Check first if there is a known defect in relatives with DVT/PE.

No useful screening method is available at present for identifying women with an increased risk of DVT/LE, but the above-mentioned investigation may be used in certain cases. If no defect has been found, there may still be a risk of DVT/PE, but at least the known risk factors have been excluded. New screening analyses are on the way.

Acquired defects

Analyze P-antithrombin, P-protein C, P-protein S free, P-APC resistance (functional method), P-lupus anticoagulant, S-cardiolipin antibodies, IgG, P-PAI-1, in addition possibly S-CRP. For physiologic changes during pregnancy see Chapter 12.

Phospholipid antibodies and lupus anticoagulant

Thromboembolic complications due to the presence of phospholipid antibodies directed against cell membrane phospholipids (e.g. cardiolipin antibodies, antibodies against phosphathidylserine and lupus anticoagulant) occur in particular in pregnancy and also secondarily to autoimmune disorders such as SLE, rheumatoid arthritis and Sjögren's syndrome, as well as in infectious diseases, above all bacterial infections (60–80% in HIV). Phospholipid antibodies lower the levels of many coagulation factors in the test systems.

Arterial thromboembolism

Analyze P-fibrinogen, P-factor VIII, P-VWF, P-PAI-1, fP-homocysteine, S-lipoprotein (a). Note, however, that the first four are also known to be acute phase reactants.

Many studies have found that high levels of the above-mentioned components are associated with arterial thromboembolism. Some have also shown high levels of FVII and the presence of phospholipid antibodies (lupus anticoagulant/cardiolipin antibodies) in arterial thromboembolism. In addition, levels of other nonhemostatic components, such as S-CRP, are high.

Disseminated intravascular coagulation

Suspected or manifest DIC

For interpretations, etc., see Chapter 14.

Indicators of the:
- *degree of hypercoagulation*: P-soluble fibrin, P-fibrin D-dimer
- *degree of consumption*: P-APT time, P-PT(INR), P-fibrinogen, B-PLT, P-antithrombin
- *degree of fibrinolysis*: P-fibrin D-dimer.

Analyze trends! New bedside methods are being introduced. See Chapter 3.

Hypercoagulation (not acute DIC)

- P-soluble fibrin, P-fibrin D-dimer.
- P-thrombin–antithrombin complex, P-prothrombin fragments 1+2 (research analyses).

Special hemostasis

PART 4

Hemostasis in obstetrics and gynecology

CHAPTER 12

Katarina Bremme

Department of Women and Child Health, Karolinska Institutet; Obstetrics and Gynecology, Karolinska University Hospital, Solna, Stockholm, Sweden

Thrombosis during pregnancy

Deep venous thrombosis (DVT) and pulmonary embolism (PE) occur in 0.5–1 out of 1000 pregnancies. The risk of DVT/PE is highest in the puerperium. Pelvic thromboses, especially on the left side, are more frequent during the later part of pregnancy and in the puerperium.

Pulmonary embolism is one of the most common causes of maternal death, with an approximate incidence of 1–2 deaths per 100,000 deliveries. The risk of lethal PE is greatest during the first few weeks post partum, especially after acute caesarean section. A higher frequency of cases of venous thromboembolism (VTE) has been reported in preeclampsia. Post-thrombotic complaints are reported in 30–60% of women with a history of deep venous thrombosis in connection with pregnancy. The risk of recurrence, especially after DVT/PE in connection with an earlier pregnancy or during treatment with contraceptives, is somewhat uncertain, but retrospective studies put it at 0–13%.

Women with hereditary or acquired thrombophilia (a biochemically verified increased risk of thrombosis, i.e. deficiencies in antithrombin, protein C or protein S, or with activated protein C (APC) resistance with or without FV Leiden mutation, with phospholipid antibodies or lupus anticoagulant) have an increased risk of DVT/PE and obstetric complications. The risk is possibly also increased in the presence of the 20210G>A polymorphism of the prothrombin gene and in hyperhomocysteinemia.

Recent data have shown that thrombophilia increases the frequency of placental thrombosis and infarction, leading to intrauterine growth

Essential Guide to Blood Coagulation. By Jovan P. Antovic and Margareta Blombäck
© Blackwell Publishing, ISBN: 9781405196277

retardation. The frequency is also increased in obstetric complications such as intrauterine embryonic death, habitual abortion, placental rejection and preeclampsia. This shows that thrombophilic factors should be investigated in women with DVT/PE, though not less than 3 months after delivery or 2 months after withdrawal of combined oral contraceptives. Reference values for nonpregnant women can be obtained not less than 1 month after the end of breastfeeding. Such an investigation (or at least analyses of antithrombin and Leiden mutation) is recommended for women with thrombophilia in first-degree relatives (parents, siblings or children) and in women with defined thrombophilia in second-degree relatives.

Diagnosis of DVT and PE during pregnancy

Suspected venous thrombosis in the leg ought to be investigated by compression ultrasonography. However, thromboses located only in the lower leg are hard to diagnose by this method, so in certain cases complementary duplex-Doppler investigation or phlebography is needed. Phlebography, with its semi-invasive character, should only be used in exceptional cases because of the iodine contrast and radiation load.

Phlebography involves relatively little radiation of the fetus, while an incorrect diagnosis can have major consequences. Table 12.1 describes the radiation dose to the fetus. A radiation dose of 0.7 mSv is comparable to the basic radiation received per year by the fetus and the lower limit when deformities can occur has been stated to be 50–150 mSv. Deformities can arise in the fetus at weeks 2–8 (organogenesis) and with regard to deformities of the CNS, at weeks 8–25.

If ultrasonography is negative and a high level of clinical suspicion exists, the patient should remain anticoagulated and ultrasonography should be repeated after 1 week or use an alternative diagnostic test. If repeated investigation is negative, stop treatment.

Computed tomography (CT) or magnetic resonance angiography (MRA) can also be considered to diagnose an isolated iliac vein thrombosis and to evaluate a vena cava thrombosis.

If a massive PE is suspected, pulmonary artery CT is performed first (without previous pulmonary X-ray in order to avoid unnecessary radiation of the fetus). Suspicion of a submassive PE leads in the first place to duplex-Doppler investigation of the legs. If thrombosis is found in the legs, further investigation of the pulmonary arteries does not affect the clinical handling.

The value of a negative D-dimer test result has not yet been assessed in pregnancy but it may possibly support a negative result in CT, ultrasonography or duplex-Doppler investigation.

Table 12.1 Calculated and estimated mean effective radiation doses to patient and fetus in radiologic investigations to diagnose VTE and for other common purposes. Individual variation may be considerable

Investigation	Effective dose to patient (mSv)	Effective dose to fetus (mSv)
Pulmonary scintigraphy		
– perfusion only	0.3	<0.1
– perfusion and ventilation	2.4	1
Pulmonary X-ray	0.1	<0.1
Pulmonary arteriography	6.6	<0.1
CT thorax	7.5	<0.1
Spiral CT thorax	2.5	<0.1
CT leg	0.8	<0.1
Phlebography (unilateral)	3.5	3
Colon	10	10
Urography	4	3
Lumbar spine	1.8	2.5
Pelvic measurement	0.5	0.5
Natural annual background radiation	1	0.7
Bone density (whole body)		0.01–0.03

Modified from SBU (Swedish Council on Technology Assessment in Health Care) report # 158/111.2002.

Women could be advised that investigation with scintigraphy carries a slightly higher risk of childhood cancer compared with CT but a lower risk of maternal breast cancer. If possible, the woman should be involved in the decision.

The choice of technique will depend on local availability. Pulmonary scintigraphy is not available in every hospital and usually not outside regular hours. Therefore CT is recommended but it also has advantages including better sensitivity and specificity and it can identify other pathology, such as aortic dissection. Thoracic CT has been reported to increase the lifetime risk of breast cancer by 14% in the mother.

In CT of the pulmonary arteries, smaller, subsegmental PE may be missed, so a negative result should be combined with ultrasonographic or duplex-Doppler investigation of the legs in order to exclude DVT/PE for certain. The fetal radiation dose is less than 10% of that with scintigraphy and therefore there is a three times lower risk of childhood cancer.

When PE exerts a hemodynamic effect, clinical evaluation is important. In massive PE, the hemodynamic effect can be evaluated by means of echocardiography.

Assay of the natriuretic peptides BNP and pro-BNP, which can now be carried out as acute tests in many hospitals, has proved to be very useful, together with determination of troponin in nonpregnant individuals, for evaluating the degree of right ventricle involvement in massive PE and the results correlate with prognosis and right ventricle involvement as determined by echocardiography.

Circulating concentrations of thyroid-stimulating hormone (TSH) ought to be assessed 1 month after investigation in all women who have undergone iodine contrast investigation. They should also be investigated in all newborn children.

Breastfeeding can continue after phlebography whether or not iodine or gadolinium contrast medium has been used, as only a negligible amount passes to the mother's milk. In lung scintillation, reduced doses of isotopes are used. There should be a pause in breastfeeding for 12 hours after the investigation.

Magnetic resonance angiography in the diagnosis of PE during pregnancy is becoming more advanced and may become the first choice. It does not require contrast medium, is independent of kidney function and contrast intolerance, and there is no irradiation. For the time being, however, MRA has not been evaluated sufficiently to support its recommendation in early pregnancy.

Treatment with anticoagulation

Unfractionated heparin (UFH) does not pass through the placenta. The need for heparin varies during pregnancy. Compared with APT time, methods used to measure anti-FXa activity are more sensitive to the anticoagulation effect of heparin. Using an anti-FXa method, it can be seen that less heparin is required to maintain a detectable anticoagulation effect. Side effects of heparin treatment are bleeding complications resulting from high doses as well as obstetric complications, and osteoporosis in long-term treatment, with vertebral fractures in about 1–2% of cases. Heparin-induced osteoporosis seems to be reversible.

Low molecular weight heparin (LMH) has many advantages over UFH. It does not pass across the placenta, is more bio-accessible and is at least as good at preventing thrombosis. It is given once a day, leads to fewer bleeding complications, a reduced risk of heparin-induced thrombocytopenia (HIT) and probably a reduced risk of osteoporosis compared with UFH. The occurrence of osteoporosis has been reported, but this can be caused by pregnancy alone. However, monitoring by means of APT time is generally not possible, as it is not sensitive enough; an anti-FXa method is required.

Antivitamin K (AVK) drugs pass through the placenta and have a teratogenic effect, primarily during pregnancy weeks 6–12. Bleeding complications can occur in both mother and fetus, but because the synthesis of coagulation factors is low in the fetus, the effect on fetal coagulation is more pronounced. Such drugs should therefore not be given during pregnancy, but might have to be considered if the need for anticoagulation therapy is extremely great, as in patients with artificial heart valves.

Treatment of acute DVT/PE during pregnancy

Blood sampling before anticoagulation treatment (with UFH/LMH) should include analyses of APT time, platelet count, PT(INR), phospholipid antibodies, lupus anticoagulant, antithrombin, protein C, protein S, homocysteine and mutation 1691G>A in the FV gene (FV Leiden) and polymorphism 20210G>A in the prothrombin gene. Sampling to test kidney and liver function is recommended in addition to analyses of hemogobin (HB), platelet count and serum homocysteine. At PT(INR) >1.2, serum creatinine >170 μmol/L, platelet count <70 × 10^9 and prolonged APT time, anticoagulation treatment should be individualized. Note that a prolonged APT time can result from the presence of lupus anticoagulant, which can increase the risk of thromboembolism.

Unfractionated heparin (5000–10,000 IU; 75 IU/kg bodyweight) is given intravenously prior to diagnostic examinations. The higher dose might be considered if PE is suspected. When DVT/PE is verified, give an intravenous continuous infusion of UFH (10,000 IU UFH/100 mL (100 U/mL) NaCl solution), usually at a drop rate of 10–20 mL/h (24,000–48,000 IU/24 h = 250 IU/kg bodyweight/12 h) (Table 12.2). However, thromboses located only in the lower leg can be treated by LMH, 10,000 IU SC twice daily, without UFH intravenously. Considering the short half-life of heparin, the infusion ought to start within an hour after the bolus dose has been given. The same infusion drop equipment should not be used for more than 12 hours owing to the risk of contamination. Twice the upper value of APT time is 70–140 sec when the reference value is 35 sec); check after 4–6 hours.

The patient should be in bed for the first 24 hours and then mobilized with a graded support stocking on the affected lower leg in the event of massive thrombosis or PE.

After 1–5 days of infusion treatment and clinical improvement, change to subcutaneous treatment twice daily with LMH: dalteparin at 125 IU/kg bodyweight, tinzaparin at 100 IU/kg bodyweight or enoxaparin at 1 mg/kg

Table 12.2 Suggestions for dosage and dilutions of heparin

	Corresponds to		Corresponds to
1 mL/h	2400 U/24 h	11 mL/h	26,400 U/24 h
2 mL/h	4800 U/24 h	12 mL/h	28,800 U/24 h
3 mL/h	7200 U/24 h	13 mL/h	31,200 U/24 h
4 mL/h	9600 U/24 h	14 mL/h	33,600 U/24 h
5 mL/h	12,000 U/24 h	15 mL/h	36,000 U/24 h
6 mL/h	14,400 U/24 h	16 mL/h	38,400 U/24 h
7 mL/h	16,800 U/24 h	17 mL/h	40,800 U/24 h
8 mL/h	19,200 U/24 h	18 mL/h	43,200 U/24 h
9 mL/h	21,600 U/24 h	19 mL/h	45,600 U/24 h

Dilute heparin to 10,000 U/100 mL NaCl.

(100 IU/kg). The level of anti-FXa should be about 0.3–0.4 IU/mL before the next injection and above 0.6 IU/mL 3 hours after an injection and should not exceed 1.3 IU/mL. The level should be checked once after 24 hours of treatment, followed by a check-up and dose adjustment once a week when a stable level has been established.

After 1 month of therapy and further clinical improvement, change to prophylactic treatment with LMH SC, twice daily (high-dose prophylaxis) in order to obtain a measurable anti-FXa concentration over 24 hours, i.e. 0.2 IU/mL before an injection and below 0.45 IU/mL 3 hours after an injection. Several centers favor a full dose treatment of LMH the whole pregnancy or three-quarters of a full dose. The latter scheme have been used for other kinds of patients with an increased bleeding risk. Therefore, test anti-FXa every second week and platelet count (PLT) once a month. Treatment should be continued until delivery. Note that the anticoagulation effect is reinforced and prolonged at the end of pregnancy, especially in high-dose treatment. Sometimes the dose may therefore need to be lowered as delivery approaches and definitely at delivery (see below).

Treatment at partus and post partum
- *If less than 1 month has passed* since the thrombotic event, reduce the LHM dose to 2500 IU every 12 hours during delivery. A vena cava filter has been used in cases with a risk of recurrence of PE and more intensive anticoagulation treatment is contraindicated.

- *If more than 1 month has passed,* you can wait for 24 hours after the last injection before the above-mentioned dosage is given. The dosage (2500 IU twice daily) is continued until the infant has been delivered.
- Antithrombin concentrate is given in cases of hereditary antithrombin deficiency or if the level of antithrombin is below 0.5 IU/mL.
- *Post partum:* AVK treatment (e.g. warfarin) starts as soon as hemostasis has been established. Use of LMH at the same dose as during the pregnancy is given for 5–7 days until the AVK treatment has a therapeutic effect. The treatment is given for at least 3 months in cases of uncomplicated lower leg thrombosis and for at least 6 months in cases of pelvic thrombosis or PE, but always for at least 6 weeks post partum. A compression stocking should be used during the day for 2 years.
- Advise the patient not to start a new pregnancy until 6–12 months after the thrombosis treatment has been completed.

Note: Oral AVK drugs, such as warfarin, are contraindicated during pregnancy, unless the patient has a mechanical heart valve prosthesis or is allergic to heparin/heparinoids and danaparoid (Orgaran) or fondaparinux (Arixtra) cannot be used (see HIT, Chapter 14). Treatment of a pregnant woman with UFH or LMH is not associated with complications in the child.

Allergy against LMH is usually evidenced as an itching redness around the injection site. In the first instance, change to another LMH drug.

After prophylactic/low-dosage LMH there does not seem to be any risk of osteoporosis. Women who have been treated with UFH or LMH at high doses should be offered investigation of bone mineral content.

Breastfeeding

Treatment with AVK, UFH or LMH does not exclude breastfeeding of fully developed children. If the child is premature the neonatologist need to be informed.

Special cases

- *Pelvic thrombosis.* Surgery, including thrombectomy and an AV fistula, has not been shown to give a better result than conventional long-term anticoagulation treatment. For circulatory disturbances in the leg, phlegmasia alba dolens, contact a vascular surgeon.
- *Massive pulmonary embolism.* Thrombolytic therapy may be indicated for a life-threatening massive PE.
- *Cerebral infarction.* Treat in consultation with a neurologist. Thrombolytic therapy may be indicated for sinus thrombosis and TIA or cerebral thrombosis (see Chapter 10).
- *Retinal thrombosis.* Treat in consultation with an ophthalmologist.

Heart disease: treatment of women with mechanical heart valve prostheses

Treatment should be given in a department with established co-operation between cardiologists, physiologists, obstetricians and coagulation experts. The mother is best protected with AVK treatment throughout the pregnancy, but in 30% of cases this will lead to pathologic consequences. Treatment with AVK in pregnancy weeks 6–12 may cause skeletal deformity (warfarin embryopathy with nasal hypoplasia and epiphysial puncture). Such treatment entails a risk of minimal brain damage throughout pregnancy, probably as a result of the bleeding risk.

Several approaches are acceptable, e.g. LMH throughout pregnancy with an adjusted dosage or LMH until the 13th week followed by AVK alone until a few weeks prior to delivery.

The decision should be influenced by patient preference. However, in very high-risk cases (older-generation prosthesis in the mitral position, history of thromboembolism or associated atrial fibrillation) we suggest AVK and a change to LMH close to delivery. All should have additional ASA (75–100 mg/day) as well as regular investigations by means of echocardiography. No data have been published on skeletal decalcification when high-dose LMH is given throughout pregnancy. Adequate protection during pregnancy may not be achieved in pregnant women with a mechanical valve.

If AVK is used, the dose should be adjusted to a target INR of 3.0 (range 2.5–3.5); the lower value can be used in a woman with an aortic valve. If LMH is used, a therapeutic value must be reached 3 hours after subcutaneous injection (>1.0 U/mL).

Active anticoagulation prophylaxis during pregnancy may be required in cyanotic heart disease.

Thromboprophylaxis in obstetrics and gynecology

Short-term prophylaxis during pregnancy is required in cases of strict immobilization, such as orthopedic immobilization (e.g. plaster) of the lower legs or that associated with major surgery and trauma. Active prophylaxis should be considered when flying (the day of the flight and the following day), if the flight lasts more than 4 hours or the woman has risk factors such as Body Mass Index over 30 kg/m^2, duplex pregnancy, thrombophilia or a clear family history of thromboembolism. Other recommendations include: exercise the legs, walk in the cabin, avoid dehydration, minimize intake of alcohol/coffee and, above all, use support stockings. Knee stockings are sufficient by themselves only for women with normal pregnancy and no risk factors. An alternative is active prophylaxis with low-dose ASA, but this is less effective than low-dose prophylaxis with dalteparin.

In thrombophilia, even without DVT/PE, always give thrombosis prophylaxis in situations associated with an increased risk of thrombosis, such as immobilization, pronounced varices, obesity, severe preeclampsia, caesarean section and complicated delivery.

In acquired thrombophilia with lupus anticoagulant established on two different occasions (with at least a 12-week interval) or with cardiolipin antibodies IgG (GPL) or IgM (MPL) at medium or high titer (>40 GPL/ MPL) established on two different occasions, or with β2-glycoprotein-1 antibody titer >99th percentile, the diagnosis is antiphospholipid syndrome (APS) together with the presence of clinical criteria such as vascular thrombosis (arterial, venous or small vessel thrombosis in any tissue or organ) or pregnancy morbidity (three or more unexplained consecutive spontaneous abortions before week 10; unexplained fetal death after week 10; delivery before week 34 because of preeclampsia or placental insufficiency). The recommended treatment is at least low-dose aspirin (LDA) besides LMH in those with earlier VTE.

Available evidence suggests that LDA during the second and third trimester is safe for the fetus and clinicians should use this agent for maternal indications. Although its safety during the first trimester remains uncertain, there is no clear evidence of harm to the fetus. If the indication is clear, clinicians should offer LDA to first-trimester patients.

Thromboprophylaxix during pregnancy, partus and post partum

- should be *considered* at partus and post partum when there is no previous DVT/PE, but thrombophilia and a clear family history of DVT/PE. Note that, in addition to antithrombin deficiency (see below), active prophylaxis may be necessary antenatally in combined or homozygous forms of prothrombin mutation 20210G>A and FV Leiden mutation, if additional risk factors are present.
- is *mandatory* at partus and postpartum for women without thrombophilia and with no family history but with earlier DVT/PE elicited by factors such as surgery, sepsis, fractures, etc.
- should be *considered* during the second and third trimesters and is *mandatory* during partus and post partum in women without thrombophilia but with earlier verified DVT/PE in connection with pregnancy or during oral contraceptive treatment or with other risk factors, such as marked obesity.
- is *mandatory* throughout pregnancy, during partus and post partum in women with:
  - ongoing DVT/PE during the current pregnancy (LMH high-dose prophylaxis)
  - ongoing treatment with AVK drugs (LMH high-dose prophylaxis)
  - inherited antithrombin deficiency (LMH high-dose prophylaxis)

- recurrent DVT/PE (LMH high-dose prophylaxis)
- DVT/PE and thrombophilia FV Leiden mutation or other thrombogenic mutations, such as prothrombin 20210G>A mutation, protein C deficiency, protein S deficiency or with phospholipid antibodies/lupus anticoagulant.

In the presence of additional risk factors, high-dose/intermediate-dose prophylaxis might be needed in combined or homozygous forms of prothrombin and Leiden mutations.

The risk of first VTE during pregnancy and the puerperium in asymptomatic double heterozygous carriers of FV Leiden and prothrombin 20210G>A is low and similar to that of single carriers. Therefore, management of pregnancy in terms of antithrombotic prophylaxis can be similar in double heterozygous and single carriers. As for single heterozygotes, antithrombotic prophylaxis in asymptomatic double heterozygous carriers appears to be justified only in the puerperium.

General comments on thromboprophylaxis

The risk of venous thromboembolism appears to arise early in pregnancy; therefore, when antepartal prophylaxis is used, it should be commenced in the first trimester.

- Coagulation analyses *before* treatment: APT time, platelet count, PT(INR), phospholipid antibodies/lupus anticoagulant and other analyses, if they have not been investigated earlier.
- Treatment with *compression stockings* starts as soon as pregnancy is apparent. This is also recommended for women with an increased risk of thrombosis without earlier DVT/PE. Compression stockings are used as early as possible in pregnancy and up to 12 weeks post partum. A knee stocking is usually sufficient. A MABS or other stocking (class I) is recommended. For chronic problems, use a class II stocking.
- Treatment with *LMH (SC)* starts in pregnancy week 16, earlier in thrombophilia and as soon as pregnancy is apparent in antithrombin-deficient women. Thrombosis prophylaxis in cases of a moderately increased risk of recurrence is given with LMH (SC), using one-dose administration (= low-dose prophylaxis) in the morning. A dose in the evening has the same effect but is not practical when blood has to be sampled. In cases of a greatly increased risk, two-dose administration (= high-dose prophylaxis) is suggested.
- In the presence of *phospholipid antibodies/lupus anticoagulant*, additional treatment with ASA should be given. Corticosteroid treatment is currently recommended only in active SLE. Folic acid should be given in hyperhomocysteinemia. (Note that levels of homocysteine normally decrease during pregnancy.) If there is no normalization, add B6 and B12 and investigate MTHFR polymorphism.

Table 12.3 Dosage of low-dose thromboprophylaxis related to body weight.

Body weight (kg) (initial weight)	Dalteparin (Fragmin) SC IU/24 h	Enoxaparin (Klexane) mg/24 h
Below 50	2500	20
50–90	5000	40
Above 90	7500	60

One of the laboratory criteria to be met is persistent lupus anti-coagulant (LA), defined as LA positivity that must be confirmed in samples 12 weeks apart. However, LA detection in patients who are under treatment with heparin and/or AVK 12 weeks later is problematic. If LMH is used for treatment, the interference is less. Note that it is important to test for LA before starting treatment.

• With previous *cerebral venous thrombosis*, LMH prophylaxis is given during pregnancy with the addition of ASA if a phospholipid antibodies/LA test is positive. Arterial cerebral thrombosis is always treated with ASA, with the addition of LMH in thrombophilia.

For a moderately increased risk, see the dosage in Table 12.3. The dosage of tinzaparin (Innohep) is given in the literature as 4500 IU anti-FXa SC × 1.

Thromboprophylaxis for women of medium weight (50–90 kg) can be given at the initial dose throughout pregnancy. If bodyweight is below 50 kg or above 90 kg, we recommend control of anti-FXa activity 3 hours *after* an injection, after 2–3 weeks of prophylaxis. The aim is an anti-FXa activity corresponding to 0.20–0.45 IU/mL. With adequate anti-FXa activity, further controls are not necessary unless there is an abnormal weight increase, or obstetric complications. Dose adjustments should be made in steps of 2500 IU/24 h and checked after 1–2 weeks. APT time and platelet count should be checked 2–3 weeks after the start of thromboprophylaxis and in pregnancy week 34.

When treated with LMH, control platelet count after 2 weeks, as HIT may occur. If platelet count is unexpectedly decreased (by 50% from baseline), see Chapter 14. Suspicion of HIT is strong if there is no other reason for the thrombocytopenia or thrombosis is increasing.

Thromboprophylaxis at birth

On arrival at the delivery department, APT time, platelet count, PT(INR) and antithrombin should be checked to evaluate the risk of bleeding and the possible need for antithrombin concentrate. Note the time of the latest injection.

In spontaneous labor, give LMH (dalteparin), 2500 IU SC 24 hours after the previous LMH dose and thereafter every 12 hours until the infant is delivered. At induction of delivery, the morning dose of LMH is reduced to 2500 IU.

After partus, give the same dose of LMH as the patient had prior to delivery, 2–4 hours after partus if no excessive bleeding is present. If bleeding is present, reduce the dosage.

Thromboprophylaxis in the puerperium

Post partum, LMH (dalteparin) SC at 5000 IU/24 h, enoxaparin at 40 mg/24 h or tinzaparin at 4500 IU/24 h is given for at least 6 weeks in the morning or evening, depending on when partus occurred. The interval after the last dose during partus should not exceed 12 hours. Monitoring by means of anti-FXa determinations is not needed unless there is an absolute indication. If prolonged thromboprophylaxis (more than 6 weeks) is planned, consider changing to AVK treatment. LMH is given until PT(INR) is 2.0–3.0 for at least 2 days and AVK treatment has been given for 5 days. Bone density measurement is recommended as soon as possible post partum after high-dose prophylaxis (two-dose) and/or simultaneous cortisone treatment. In extended osteopenia, consider continued thromboprophylaxis with AVK and follow-up of bone density 1 year after delivery. Refer to an endocrinologist thereafter if needed.

With a greatly increased risk, two-dose prophylaxis (= high-dose prophylaxis) should be used.

For all other pregnant women with thrombophilia and no prior VTE, antepartal clinical surveillance is suggested plus postpartal anticoagulants. At present, complete thrombophilia investigation is carried out. If the father has a family history of thrombosis, he ought to be investigated with regard to thrombophilic factors.

Thromboprophylaxis in antithrombin deficiency

Thromboprophylaxis should start as early as possible in pregnancy. A measurable anticoagulation effect in 24 hours is desired. Dalteparin is given at 5000–7500 IU SC twice daily with an anti-FXa level of 0.1–0.2 U/mL immediately prior to the injection. Anti-FXa should be checked every second week and, during the last 2 months, every week.

During delivery, in early puerperium and with obstetric complications, we recommend normalizing the inhibitory capacity with antithrombin concentrate. An adequate dose of antithrombin (AT) is calculated in IU as follows: (a) kg × (desired AT level minus the current AT level, both in IU/mL) × 100, or (b) kg × (desired AT level minus the current AT level, both in %). Desired level: 1.0–1.4 IU/mL or 100–140%.

When the antithrombin level has been normalized, the dose of dalteparin can be reduced. In view of the risk of bleeding, when treatment with antithrombin concentrate is combined with high-dose LMH, treatment with AVK drugs can wait until a couple of days after partus. During the following week, the antithrombin concentration in plasma should exceed 80%. Prophylactic anticoagulation treatment should continue for 3 months post partum, or for longer if the woman has had an earlier DVT/PE.

The infant should be investigated after birth for antithrombin deficiency and treated on suspicion of hereditary antithrombin deficiency.

Ongoing treatment with AVK drugs and with recurrent DVT/PE in anamnesis

If the patient is on AVK treatment (warfarin, etc.), we recommend planning pregnancy in advance so that when a test confirms the pregnancy, a change to LMH can be made *before* pregnancy week 6. Note that AVK must be withdrawn.

Thromboprophylaxis should start as early as possible in the pregnancy. A measurable anticoagulation effect in 24 hours is desirable. Give dalteparin at 5000–7500 IU SC twice daily, aiming for an anti-FXa level of 0.1–0.2 U/mL immediately prior to an injection. Anti-FXa should be monitored every month up to week 32, every second week up to the last month, and during the last month, every week.

If anti-FXa is below 0.1 U/mL, increase the evening dose in the first place by 2500 IU dalteparin or by 20 mg enoxaparin respectively.

On arrival at the delivery department, check APT time, PT(INR), antithrombin and platelet count. Note the time of the last LMH injection. In order to make regional anesthesia possible in spontaneous labor, wait for 24 hours and thereafter reduce the LMH dose to half, twice daily. For instance, reduce the dalteparin dose to 2500 IU/mL twice daily. Women treated with low-dose ASA due to acquired thrombophilia, SLE nephritis or stroke should remain on this.

On induction/caesarean section, omit the evening dose to prepare for regional anesthesia/catheterization in the morning. High-dose prophylaxis should be resumed as soon as possible after postoperative supervision. Women on AVK prior to pregnancy can resume this treatment 1–2 days after delivery, but it may be an advantage to wait for 2–3 weeks and continue with high-dose LMH instead.

Thromboprophylaxis at caesarean section

A thrombosis risk assessment should be performed in all women undergoing caesarean section to determine the need for thromboprophylaxis.

The risk of thromboembolism in an elective caesarean section is low in an uncomplicated pregnancy with no risk factors and similar to that seen in low-risk surgical patients for whom no routine thromboprophylaxis other than early mobilization is recommended. Support stockings are recommended. Routine thromboprophylaxis is not justified and cannot be recommended on the basis of caesarean section alone.

Prophylaxis with LMH should be considered for a moderate risk of thromboembolism with risk factors such as acute caesarean section, older age (>35 years), obesity (BMI >30 kg/m^2), multiparae (four or more), pronounced varices, ongoing infection, preeclampsia, immobilization, immobility for >4 days prior to surgery, large amount of blood loss, dehydration, sickle cell anemia, inflammatory intestinal disorder or nephrotic syndrome and other co-morbid medical conditions such as heart failure.

The presence of three risk factors represents a high risk and thromboprophylaxis must be given. A high risk also exists with simultaneous hysterectomy, hereditary thrombotic disease, paralysis of the lower legs and in the presence of phospholipid antibodies/lupus anticoagulant.

For thromboprophylaxis, dalteparin (5000 IU × 1) should be given until the fifth postoperative day or until full mobilization. The first injection is given 2–4 hours after the operation. Prophylaxis for 6–12 weeks post partum may be indicated if risk factors such as thrombophilia are still present.

Thromboprophylaxis at vaginal delivery

Prophylaxis to cover delivery should not be limited to those undergoing caesarean section. Age >35 years and BMI >30 kg/m^2 are important independent risk factors of postpartum VTE even after vaginal delivery. The combination of either of these risk factors with any other risk factor of VTE (preeclampsia, immobility or inflammatory disorders) justifies the use of LMH for 3–5 days post partum. Women who qualify for post-partum LMH prophylaxis can probably safely discontinue this after 3–5 days if they are fully mobile.

Blood sampling in children of women with severe forms of thrombophilia

The father should be analyzed with regard to the same deficiency that the mother has and asked about a family history of thromboembolism.

In antithrombin deficiency analyze the AT level at the same time as investigation of phenylketonuria (PKU) if the child is otherwise healthy. After a traumatic delivery or if the child is affected, analyze AT immediately and contact a coagulation expert for discussion about treatment with antithrombin concentrate. Avoid use of any remaining IV ingoing catheter. Carry out ultrasonographic investigation of the head of a child with a decreased AT level.

Analyze AT level again at the age of 6 months.

If the woman has a deficiency of protein C or protein S, the child is sampled at the same time as for PKU.

Obstetric epidural/spinal analgesia (anethesia)

In low-dose prophylaxis with LMH, epidural anesthesia (EDA) can be used when APT time, PT(INR) and platelet count are normal and at least 10 hours have passed since the injection of 5000 IU dalteparin or 40 mg enoxaparin given as a single dose. If only LMH (2500 IU SC) has been given after the beginning of labor, the time from injection to EDA/spinal anesthesia can be reduced, but it must be at least 6 hours. The next prophylactic dose can be given 2 hours after EDA/spinal anesthesia at the earliest. The catheter is removed 10 and 6 hours, respectively, after the last injection. A new injection is given at the earliest 2 hours after EDA if the catheter is still in place.

In high-dose prophylaxis and treatment
In high-dose prophylaxis with a two-dose regime or treatment dosage, 24 hours must have passed since the latest injection before EDA/spinal analgesia can be allowed. Accumulation is to be expected in high-dose prophylaxis/treatment, so the anti-FXa level must be measured *exactly* as close to delivery if possible. When anti-FXa activity is known, EDA may be considered earlier if the trough value is below 0.1 U/mL.

In ASA medication (75–160 mg)
Trombyl® (ASA) medication should, if possible, be discontinued 2–3 days prior to planned EDA. If this is not advisable EDA can still be performed provided no other risk factors are present.

In platelet function deficiency
In platelet function deficiency, EDA/spinal anesthesia can be used if bleeding time is normal (tested within 1 week). APT time, PT(INR) and platelet count should be normal. Spinal anesthesia for section can be performed if the bleeding time is only slightly prolonged (up to 600 s measured as template bleeding time with a reference value below 420 s). Spinal anesthesia is preferable in this situation. Epidural anesthesia should not be performed as a pain reliever in vaginal delivery if bleeding time is prolonged. Desmopressin treatment to make spinal anesthesia possible before section should not be carried out routinely. Consult coagulation and anesthesia specialists and an obstetrician.

In preeclampsia
In preeclampsia, EDA/spinal anesthesia can be performed if platelet count is above 100×10^9/L. It is not necessary to control APT time and PT(INR) routinely. With platelet count at $80–100 \times 10^9$/L, EDA/spinal anesthesia can be considered if APT time, PT(INR) and bleeding time

are normal. How early in advance the samples have to be drawn is often debated. This has to be considered from case to case. Mostly it is acceptable with samples drawn the same day, but sometimes it is necessary to draw and analyze samples just before the anesthesia.

In ITP, the same applies as in preeclampsia.

In VWD

In many cases of VWD, EDA/spinal anesthesia is contraindicated. In patients with mild VWD type 1, when the levels of VWF have increased to >0.70 kIU/L during pregnancy, EDA/spinal anesthesia can be used if APT time, PT(INR), platelet count and bleeding time are normal at the same time. These analyses are carried out in the third trimester and it is not necessary to repeat them routinely. The level of VWF decreases quickly after delivery and therefore a remaining epidural catheter ought to be removed 2 hours after partus (i.e. as in normal delivery).

In carriers of hemophilia A or B

Epidural/spinal anesthesia can be used if the levels of FVIII and FIX are >0.70 kIU/L and at the same time APT time, PT(INR), platelet count and bleeding time are normal. These analyses are carried out in the third trimester/week 32 and need not be repeated thereafter.

In antiphospholipid syndrome, SLE

If a prolonged APT time is due to the presence of LA, no further coagulation investigation is needed. If no LA is found, investigation of coagulation factors has to be carried out. However, planning before EDA/spinal anesthesia has to be carried out in all cases with prolonged APT time, together with a coagulation specialist. A necessary prerequisite before using EDA is that the woman has no bleeding history.

Complications during pregnancy

The hemostatic balance changes during pregnancy in order to prevent bleeding at delivery. Levels of most coagulation factors increase and fibrinolytic capability decreases (see Tables 12.4 and 12.5).

Hemophilia, VWD

During a normal pregnancy, FVIII roughly doubles and VWF increases up to fourfold. The factor levels should be measured in pregnancy week 32 in hemophilia A carriers (FVIII) and in severe and mild VWD (VWF). Factor IX is not elevated at the end of pregnancy, so hemophilia B carriers might have a higher risk of bleeding.

Table 12.4 Hemostatic variables (indices) during normal pregnancy

Variable	Pregnancy week			Delivery	5 weeks Post-partum	Breast-feeding	Ref. values
	12–15	24	35	(n = 16)	(n = 19)	(n = 12–14)	
B-platelet count (×10⁹/L)	275±64	256±49	244±52	246±54	243±61	267±57	150–400
P-fibrinogen (g/L)	3.7±0.6	4.4±1.2	5.4±0.8	5.7±0.7	3.1±0.7	3.1±1.0	2.1–4.2
P-PT (%)*	120±27	140±27	130±27	144±30	102±8.7	90±18	70–130
P-antithrombin (IU/mL)	1.02±0.10	1.07±0.14	1.07±0.11	1.06±0.14	1.09±0.16	1.08±0.12	0.85–1.25
P-protein C (U/mL)	0.92±0.13	1.06±0.17	0.94±0.2	1.01±0.20	1.03±0.14	0.91±0.17	0.68–1.25
P-protein S, total (U/mL)	0.83±0.11	0.73±0.11	0.77±0.10	0.77±0.11	0.93±0.11	1.00±0.18	0.70–1.70
P-protein S, free (U/mL)	0.26±0.07	0.17±0.04	0.14±0.04	0.12±0.05	0.19±0.06	0.25±0.06	0.20–0.50
P-fibrin, soluble (nmol/L)	9.2±8.6	11.8±7.7	13.4±5.2	17.2±13.9	9.4±4.4	9.7±6.2	<15
P-TAT (µg/L)	3.1±1.4	5.9±2.6	7.1±2.4	8.2±2.5	1.9±0.5	2.1±0.7	<2.7
P-fibrin D-dimer (µg/L)	91±24	128±49	198±59	266±101	84±14	81±34	<80
P-PAI-1 (AU/mL)	7.4±4.9	14.9±5.2	37.8±19.4	33.3±14.5	6.0±3.1	8.1±4.9	<15
P-PAI-2 (µg/L)	31±14	84±16	160±31	150±45	3.0±8.7	1.3±1.9	<5
S-cardiolipin antibodies pos. results	2/25	2/25	3/23	2/16	2/11		0

* For transformation to INR see www.equalis.se – INR. See Chapter 3.

From Bremme *et al. Obstet Gynecol* 1992:**80:**132–137.

P, plasma; TAT, thrombin–antithrombin complex; PAI, plasminogen activator inhibitor. Data are presented as mean ± SD. Unless otherwise indicated, 24–26 women were investigated during pregnancy.

Table 12.5 Some coagulation factors at different stages of pregnancy
(mean ± 95% ranges). n = 60

	Week of pregnancy			8 w post partum	Breastfeeding
	11–15	21–25	31–35		
Factor VII	111 (60–206)	150 (80–280)	162 (84–312)	94	91
Factor X	103 (62–69)	115 (74–177)	123 (78–194)	91	92
Factor V	93 (46–188)	82 (36–185)	82 (34–195)	80	84
Factor II*	125 (70–224)	125 (73–214)	115 (74–179)	106	107
FVIII:C	122 (53–833)	141 (44–453)	185 (69–499)	86	109
VWF	133 (56–318)	167 (66–427)	262 (95–718)	93	78

Modified from Stirling *et al. Thromb Haemost* 1984;**52**:176–182.
* Prothrombin.
Comment: VWF increases about fourfold and FVIII:C doubles.

Hemophilia A and B and severe forms of VWD are rare. Written recommendations concerning pregnancy and delivery are issued by the doctor in charge of the delivery in co-operation with the coagulation specialist. In hemophilia, ultrasonographic determination of the sex of the fetus is recommended. Section is not indicated routinely, only for a complicated or prolonged delivery. Vacuum extraction and scalp electrodes should be avoided. An umbilical cord test in infant boys with suspected or known hemophilia (analyses of FVIII/FIX) is recommended.

For treatment of severe forms of hemophilia, see Chapter 4.

Carriers of mild VWD and hemophilia are treated with tranexamic acid (Cyklokapron 500 mg, 3 tablets 3 times daily; if not per os, give IV at 10 mg/kg bodyweight) at the onset of labor, during delivery and at least 1 week post partum. For abnormal bleeding after delivery, give desmopressin; be careful about repeating doses because of the possibility of electrolytic disturbances (see Chapter 4).

Idiopathic thrombocytopenia purpura

Assessment of platelet count is carried out initially in both EDTA and citrate tubes. For platelet count below 100×10^9/L, investigate the presence of hematologic malignancy together with a hematologist. Because isolated thrombocytopenia is present in SLE, at least the presence of LA and cardiolipin antibodies should be determined, and the development of preeclampsia should be taken into consideration. platelet count in the mother should be followed during pregnancy.

If the woman does not have any symptoms and the number of platelets is above 50×10^9/L, there is no need for treatment during pregnancy or delivery.

Monitoring during pregnancy
- At platelet count >150×10^9/L, monitor every second month.
- At platelet count $100–150 \times 10^9$/L, monitor each month.
- At platelet count $50–100 \times 10^9$/L, monitor every second week.
- At platelet count <50×10^9/L, monitor each week.

There is probably no risk of spontaneous bleeding until platelet count is $10–20 \times 10^9$/L.

Treatment during pregnancy
Treatment during pregnancy should be considered if the platelet count is <20×10^9/L or there are bleeding complications. A platelet count >50×10^9/L is aimed at, and before delivery/caesarean section, if possible >100×10^9/L.

Intravenous immunoglobulin 0.4 g/kg/day for 3 days; alternatively 0.8–1 g for 1–2 days; effect within 1–3 days. There are few side effects.

If treated with prednisolone at 1 mg/kg/day for 7–10 days, the effect is slowly established but there are many side effects.

In treatment failure and platelet count >10×10^9/L, splenectomy can be considered on vital indication.

Fibrinolytic inhibitor, tranexamic acid, can be given prophylactically at platelet count <100×10^9/L.

Delivery
In the event of bleeding or a bleeding tendency in connection with delivery, platelet transfusions may be necessary. One unit, 300 mL, can be expected to increase platelet count by about 10×10^9/L. The effect does not last long (hours) so platelet concentrate should be given shortly before a planned operation.

An umbilical cord test (cordocentesis) is not usually recommended.

Check platelet count, APT time and PT(INR) on admission to the delivery unit. Caesarean section should be performed according to obstetric indications. Bleeding complications in the child have not been proven to be related to the manner of delivery. Fetal thrombocytopenia, however, cannot be excluded. Avoid prolonged delivery and traumatic extraction. EDA can be used if platelet count is >100×10^9/L and spinal anesthesia if platelet count is >80×10^9/L. The risk of neonatal thrombocytopenia is greatest during the first few days after delivery.

The newborn infant

Circulating antibodies can cross the placenta during pregnancy and give rise to thrombocytopenia. ITP is not hereditary but it is important to inform the mother during pregnancy about the risk of transient thrombocytopenia in the child. Assess platelet count in the umbilical cord blood. A neonatology specialist should be informed and give an opinion about the platelet count after delivery and during the first 24 hours. Platelet counts should be monitored for 3 days and possible treatment with immunoglobulin should be given. The platelet level becomes normalized during the first few months.

Essential thrombocytosis (ET; thrombocythaemia)

The clinical course of ET is most often benign in the young. It should be remembered that around 85% of cases of thrombocytosis are reactive (bleeding, iron deficiency, malignancy, connective disease, splenectomy) rather than primary phenomena. Women with essential thrombocytosis have an increased risk of complications during pregnancy, possibly related to placental thromboses. However, platelet count can decrease during pregnancy. If platelet count is above $600 \times 10^9/L$, we recommend low-dose ASA medication. Cytostatics should be avoided during pregnancy, but interferon can be used for myelosuppression.

Preeclampsia

For women with preeclampsia, the risk of the condition is increased tenfold in the next pregnancy and is even higher if a previous pregnancy was associated with a medical risk factor or early/severe preeclampsia. Preeclampsia can occur without a clear cause but mainly if the woman develops high blood pressure.

For women with earlier severe or repeated preeclampsia, ablation, intrauterine growth retardation (IUGR) or unexplained intrauterine fetal death (IUFD), we recommend screening for hereditary thrombophilia, phospholipid antibodies and hyperhomocysteinemia.

Thrombophilia is not the cause of preeclampsia but it contributes to the disease.

Placental ablation, severe preeclampsia and HELLP syndrome (Hemolysis, Elevated Liver enzymes, Low Platelet counts) can cause severe disseminated intravascular coagulation (DIC). Total ablation is always accompanied by some form of coagulopathy. Coagulation disturbances in IUFD are rare, but control of platelet count, fibrinogen and antithrombin is recommended before partus. If an acquired hemostasis disturbance is suspected, check on platelet count, APTT, PT(INR), antithrombin and fibrin D-dimer, with an additional test of fibrinogen in case of bleeding. Nowadays, thromboelastography (TEG) can give a complete picture of hemostatic function (platelet function, coagulation and fibrinolysis).

Soluble fibrin, reflecting formation of thrombin, can be used to detect DIC at an early stage. In pregnancy, fibrin D-dimer analysis and balance methods are useful (see Chapters 3 and 14).

Acute fatty liver of pregnancy

This is a rare condition almost always seen during third trimester of pregnancy. Acute fatty liver of pregnancy is characterized by malaise, nausea, epigatric pain and sometimes changes in mental status. Laboratory studies show moderate to severe abnormal liver function tests, hypoglycemia and electrolyte imbalance. Coagulopathy ensues due to depressed clotting factor synthesis. Although the diagnosis of AFLP can be made clinically, confirmation can be achieved by a liver biopsy.

Treatment should be aggressive in order to deliver as soon as possible.

Thrombotic thrombocytopenia purpura (TTP)

This is a rare disease characterized by a triad of microangiopathic hemolytic anemia (fragmented RBC in smears and elevated LDH), thrombocytopenia and neurologic symptoms. The etiology has recently been shown to be due to severe deficiency of a VWF-cleaving protease, ADAMTS13. Two clinical forms have been described – acquired deficiency and congenital. The apparent higher incidence of TTP in pregnancy appears to be due to an overlap of a TTP-like syndrome with HUS, HELLP and severe preeclampsia.

Prophylaxis against preeclampsia

General prophylaxis against preeclampsia with ASA has not proved to be of any value, except possibly in cases of early onset of severe preeclampsia (causing delivery prior to pregnancy week 34). However, studies have shown that low-dose ASA can be used without risk during pregnancy. For women considered to be at high risk of preeclampsia, low-dose ASA throughout pregnancy is recommended. It is therefore reasonable to give 75 mg ASA daily as prophylaxis to women with high blood pressure and either kidney disorders or diabetes, or antiphospholipid syndrome, and especially to women with early-onset or severe or repeated preeclampsia.

In patients with earlier severe preeclampsia with elective delivery or IUFD before week 34 and microvascular events in the woman (usually in the kidney or cerebral) and phospholipid antibodies (especially in the presence of LA and high levels of cardiolipin antibodies or b2-glycoprotein-1), a high-dosage prophylaxis program together with ASA is mandatory. When using ASA, treatment should start in or before pregnancy week 12. Further studies are needed to confirm the usefulness of treatment with folic acid (5 mg/day), vitamin C (1000 mg/day) and vitamin E (400 IU/day) in high-risk populations.

The level of plasminogen activator inhibitor-1 (PAI-1), normally present in the blood, is increased in preeclampsia and is connected with increased resistance in the placental circulation. Plasminogen activator inhibitor-2 (PAI-2) forms in the placenta and is not present in the blood except during pregnancy. The level of PAI-2 in the mother is significantly correlated to placental function and weight and also to fetal growth, but it is not correlated to the severity of preeclampsia. Intrauterine growth inhibition is accompanied by reduced fibrinolysis, measured as lower levels of fibrin D-dimer compared with women with preeclampsia but no fetal growth inhibition. Levels of fibrin D-dimer are, however, higher than in healthy pregnant women.

Fibronectin has not been shown to be suitable for screening, although it probably indicates a pathologic development earlier than does elevated blood pressure. Besides fibronectin soluble Flt-1, control of angiogenes, is shown to increase five weeks prior to to the onset of preeclampsia and an increased ratio of sFlt-1/PlGF ratio strongly predicts the future onset of preeclampsia. The cytokine TNF-alfa is a strong candidate for mediating endothelial damage as recent reports suggest that serum concentrations are significantly higher already in the first trimester in pregnant women who go on to develop preeclampsia compared to controls.

Postpartum bleeding

The volume of blood in a highly pregnant woman is 5–6 liters. Blood flow in the spiral arteries increases to 600–800 mL/min at term.

A clinically massive loss of blood is defined as 50% of the total volume in 3 hours, or 150 mL/min. Blood loss equivalent to the total volume of the patient results in dilution of the platelet concentration to 40–50% of the original; after the loss of 1.5–2 blood volumes, the concentration of fibrinogen in the blood can fall below 1 g/L and PT(INR) can rise above 1.5.

General procedures
Act promptly.
- Search for a local source of bleeding – first surgery and arterial ligation.
- Keep the patient warm, calm and free from pain.
- Take samples for INR, platelet counts (PLT), APT time, fibrinogen, D-dimer and AT.
- Independently of the response from the laboratory, promptly administer tranexamic acid 10–20 mg/kg bodyweight IV. Dosage 3–4 times/24 h IV in normal kidney function.
- If after 5 minutes massive bleeding continues, give 2–4 g of fibrinogen concentrate. An ampoule containing 1 g fibrinogen increases the concentration by 0.3 g/L.

- Thereafter give fresh-frozen plasma 15 mL/kg bodyweight and consider giving platelet concentrate.
- Prothrombin complex concentrate can be used if plasma treatment fails to have sufficient effect on PT(INR).
- If bleeding still continues, consider giving antithrombin concentrate if the level of antithrombin is <0.50 IU/L and platelet concentrate if platelet count <50 × 10⁹.
- The indication for transfusion at ongoing bleeding is HB > 100 but if the situation is stabilized at HB > 80.
- Give LMH when bleeding is under control.

Recombinant factor VIIa Novoseven is being increasingly proposed for massive bleeding despite a lack of clinical studies on its effect and safety. However, its use has also been associated with thromboembolic complications (see also Chapter 5).

Consider using NovoSeven:

- for blood loss of 1.5 times the total volume
- when considering hysterectomy, so that extirpation of the uterus may be avoided
- when planning selective embolization, so that embolism can be delayed or avoided.

Prior to administration of NovoSeven, the following should be fulfilled: hemoglobin concentration above 70 g/L, PT(INR) above 1.5, platelet count above 50 × 10⁹/L, fibrinogen above 2.0 g/L, pH above 7.1.

If laboratory results are not known, give two units of platelet concentrate and fresh (frozen) plasma (10–20 mL/kg body weight).

Dosage of NovoSeven: give 0.1 mg/kg as an IV bolus over 2–3 minutes (7 mg to a 70 kg patient – round off upwards). Combine this with tranexamic acid (10–20 mg/kg bodyweight). If there is no effect within 15–30 min., repeat the dose *once*.

Thromboprophylaxis in legal and spontaneous abortions

If the patient is in need of thrombosis prophylaxis during pregnancy but wants a legal abortion for medical or social reasons, LMH (dalteparin 5000 IU SC × 1) should be given as soon as possible. The medication should continue for 1–2 weeks after abortion.

For spontaneous or threatened miscarriage, the dose can be adjusted to 2500 IU twice daily.

Thromboprophylaxis in gynecologic surgery

The surgeon in charge decides which patient should have thrombosis prophylaxis and notes the prescription in the drug record on arrival. Indications include the following.

- All patients over 40 years of age undergoing laparotomy or similar operations.
- All patients regardless of age undergoing laparotomy or similar operations because of a malignant disease.
- All patients regardless of age having a reoperation within 30 days.
- Risk factors that, regardless of age, should be taken into account as regards laparatomy and similar operations:
  - earlier thromboembolic disease
  - obesity (BMI above 30 kg/m^2)
  - extensive varices
  - long operation (more than 90 minutes)
  - ongoing medication with oral contraceptives or HRT
  - pregnancy.

Prophylaxis consists of the following.

- *LMH* (dalteparin, 5000 IU), anti-FXa SC × 1, or enoxaparin (40 mg SC × 1) is given, starting in the evening prior to the operation day. The treatment should continue for at least 5 days or for longer if immobilization continues. With a high risk of bleeding, the dose can be halved.
- *Dextran60 + LMH*. Dextran60 (1000 mL) is given preoperatively after 20 mL Dextran1 to a patient who has not had LMH the previous evening. Postoperatively, LMH is given as above, starting on the first day after the operation.
- *Dextran60 alone*. The patient is given 1000 mL Dextran60 after 20 mL Dextran1 during the operation and possibly on the first day after the operation.

Low molecular weight heparin is the first alternative in elective operations. Dextran60 alone is suitable in most acute operations and in those with a low risk, e.g. in vaginal hysterectomy in a healthy woman over 40 years of age.

Oral contraceptives, hormone substitution

In cases of sizeable elective surgery leading to immobilization, contraceptive (p-pills) treatment should be discontinued 4–6 weeks prior to surgery and started 4–6 weeks after surgery. Inform the patient about advantages and disadvantages and also about alternative contraceptive methods.

For acute surgery or elective surgery while contraceptives are still in use, for plastering of lower-leg fractures and for long-term immobilization, thrombosis prophylaxis with LMH should be given. Women with hormone substitution already have additional risk factors indicating thrombosis prophylaxis.

Investigation before oral contraceptives, advice concerning oral contraceptives

For women 15–44 years old who are not on oral contraceptives that contain estrogen, the risk of DVT/PE is 5–10 cases/100,000 women-years. The second generation of oral contraceptives increases the risk to 20 cases/ 100,000 women-years and the third generation entails a further increase. The most serious complication is PE, present in 10% of these cases and fatal in 1–2%. This should be taken into consideration when oral contraceptives containing estrogen are prescribed for the first time, because for all combined oral contraceptives, the risk of thrombosis is greatest during the first year.

No screening method is yet available for adequate identification of women at risk prior to or during the use of oral contraceptives, even though 25–40% of the women who develop thrombosis are APC resistant (most of them have the FV Leiden mutation). Combined oral contraceptives are associated with a decreased sensitivity to APC, in certain cases to such an extent that the woman develops so-called acquired APC resistance. This type of APC resistance also carries an increased risk of venous thrombosis.

For women with earlier thrombosis, combined oral contraceptives are contraindicated. Nowadays, many of these women have undergone coagulation investigation.

Women who have a first-degree relative with thrombosis are advised to avoid oral contraceptives containing estrogen regardless of what coagulation investigation shows. Even women with several second-degree relatives should be advised to avoid oral contraceptives.

Women with a known heterozygous form of APC resistance should avoid oral contraceptives containing estrogen, and for those with a homozygous form they should not be used. In hereditary thrombophilia, such as antithrombin deficiency, oral contraceptives should not be given, neither should they be given to women with acquired thrombophilia, such as lupus anticoagulant or significantly increased levels of cardiolipin antibodies.

Women with a strong fear of thrombosis should choose a contraceptive that does not contain estrogen. These women can of course undergo coagulation investigations, but what matters most is a thorough anamnesis and good information.

For most women with medical disorders, pregnancy is associated with risks other than the use of oral contraceptives.

Methods other than combined (estrogen-progesterone) contraceptives (p-pills) should be considered in women as regards the following:
• age over 35 years and a smoker

- migraine headache and co-existing vascular risk factors, vascular disease or age over 35 years
- earlier thromboembolic disease
- coronary disease
- cerebrovascular disease
- chronic liver disease
- less than 3 weeks after delivery in a nonbreastfeeding woman (an intrauterine device is not suitable up to 6 weeks after delivery)
- diabetes mellitus with vascular disease or age over 35 years
- SLE and vascular disease, nephritis or phospholipid antibodies
- hypertriglyceridemia.

In the above-mentioned women, a contraceptive containing progesterone or a copper/hormone intrauterine device is safer than combined contraceptives. At present there are no scientific indications that contraceptives containing gestagens only increase the risk of venous or arterial thrombosis.

Acute oral contraceptives (p-pills)

When acute p-pills (day-after pills) are administered, a high dose of steroid hormones (gestagen or a combination with estrogen) is given in a very short time. The risk of thrombosis has been investigated in just a few studies, none of which shows any risk of DVT/PE. There are no contraindications for acute p-pills that contain only gestagen, so these drugs can be chosen for women with an increased risk of thrombosis.

Investigation prior to postclimacteric substitution treatment

The risk of DVT/PE increases with age and for postmenopausal women it is approximately twice as high as for premenopausal women. Investigate anamnesis in the event of thromboembolic disease in first- or second-degree relatives. HRT increases the risk during the first year. This information should be given when prescribing HRT. Routine screening for thrombophilia is not indicated. HRT should be avoided in women with multiple DVT/LE risk factors in anamnesis.

There is no epidemiologic evidence that parenteral HRT is more advantageous than oral HRT, though comparative studies have shown that parenteral HRT leads to fewer effects on coagulation. Oral HRT should not be given to patients with earlier thrombosis with or without hereditary thrombophilia.

In women who have had DVT/PE, stroke/TIA or with a close family history of such conditions, an investigation of thrombophilia might improve the assessment of risk. In those with no thrombosis but with known thrombophilia, HRT should be avoided in cases of antithrombin deficiency or a finding of several combined thrombophilias.

There are no epidemiologic studies, but published data indicate that regarding the risk of thrombosis, parenteral (transdermal or vaginal) hormone is safer than oral. Separate studies have shown that parenteral administration has less effect on coagulation inhibitors and it entails a loss of coagulation activation.

Selective estrogen receptor modulators (SERM), such as raloxifen and tamoxifen, have antiestrogenic effects on breast tissue and uterine mucous membranes, but they affect hemostasis in the same way as estrogens.

If DVT/PE develops during HRT, the HRT must be withdrawn. If the woman wishes to remain on HRT, prolonged anticoagulation therapy should be considered.

Investigation prior to artificial insemination

The brief hormonal stimulation probably adds somewhat to the risk of thrombosis. If the patient has had earlier thrombosis or high risk for VTE, it is reasonable to give thrombosis prophylaxis with LMH (dalteparin 5000 IU SC × 1) at the start of the hormone treatment. At sign of over-stimulation it is reasonable to start prophylaxis and continue two weeks after normalisation.

Investigation in repeated miscarriages

Repeated miscarriages occur in 1% of all women. Thrombophilia is widespread in women who have had repeated miscarriages, above all in those who have never given birth (primary miscarriers). About 15–25% of women with three or more miscarriages are found to have phospholipid antibody syndrome. The most common hereditary thrombophilia is caused by the FV Leiden mutation, which is present in about 28% of women with primary miscarriage.

Investigation of women with repeated miscarriages should include assessment of cardiolipin antibodies, β2-glycoprotein-1, lupus anticoagulant, FV Leiden mutation, prothrombin mutation, protein S, protein C, antithrombin and homocysteine.

In patients with repeated miscarriages and phospholipid antibodies, treatment with low-dose ASA increases the probability of having a live-born child from 10% to 40%. Combined treatment with ASA and low-dose LMH increases this probability to 70%. Especially in the group with one or more cases of unexplained death of a normal fetus at or beyond the 10th week of gestation (late miscarriage), treatment with LMH should be considered. The pregnancies are still high risk, with complications during all trimesters, miscarriages, preeclampsia and inhibited growth, despite treatment and close supervision. Ongoing studies are aimed at clarifying treatment of miscarriage propensity in other thrombophilias.

For women with Leiden mutations and earlier placental thrombosis, there is a case for thrombosis prophylaxis.

Women with an inexplicable propensity for miscarriage have a good prognosis in future pregnancies without pharmacologic intervention if TLC (tender loving care) is provided!

Investigation in menorrhagia (for treatment see Chapter 4)

Menorrhagia is experienced by 10–20% of women of fertile age. A number of studies indicate that this group has an increased frequency of a mild hemostatic defect, above all VWD type 1, and platelet function disorders.

Investigation of suspected coagulation disturbances include, in the first place, blood status, APT time, PT(INR), CRP, bleeding time, platelet count, FVIII and VWF analyses (state blood group). Sampling should be carried out during cycle days 1–4, if possible.

Note that a levonorgestrel-releasing intrauterine system decreases menstrual bleeding by up to 97%.

Hemostasis defects in children

CHAPTER 13

Pia Petrini

Department of Women and Child Health, Karolinska Institutet; Pediatrics Department, Karolinska University Hospital, Solna, Stockholm, Sweden

Bleeding disorders in children

The hemostasis system, i.e. endothelial function and coagulation and fibrinolysis factors are influenced by age. Though the hemostasis system is considered to be "immature" in children, it is functionally adequate, i.e. bleeding or thrombosis is rare in healthy full-term newborns. The morbidity, however, can be affected in prematurely born or severely ill newborns.

The synthesis of coagulation factors starts during the first trimester of pregnancy and increases successively with the gestation age of the fetus. Consequently, the measured levels of these proteins in plasma should be related to prenatal as well as postnatal age. The tables (13.1 and 13.2) show reference values for some of these proteins in relation to age of the child. These proteins do *not* pass from the mother via the placenta to the fetus.

At birth, concentrations of the vitamin K-dependent coagulation factors (FII, FVII, FIX, FX) and FXI and FXII are about 50% of adult values. Also, levels of the coagulation inhibitors antithrombin, protein C and protein S are reduced. Because of this, both the formation and inhibition of thrombin are reduced in newborns. This is considered to be one of the factors contributing to the reduced risk of developing a thrombosis in children. The levels of FV, FVIII, FXIII and von Willebrand factor (VWF) are the same at birth as in adults, or elevated. Also, the fibrinolysis system differs in newborns with low plasminogen levels but increased levels of t-PA and PAI-1. The hemostasis system matures during the first months of life. The

Essential Guide to Blood Coagulation. By Jovan P. Antovic and Margareta Blombäck
© Blackwell Publishing, ISBN: 9781405196277

Table 13.1 Hemostasis variables in full-term children during the first 6 months compared with adults

Variable	Day 1	Day 5	Day 30	Day 90	Day 180	Adults
Fibrinogen g/L	2,83 (1,67–3,99)	3,12 (1,62–4,62)*	2,70 (1,62–3,78)*	2,43 (1,50–3,79)*	2,51 (1,50–3,87)*	2,78 (1,56–4,00)
Prothrombin (U/mL)	0,48 (0,26–0,70)	0,63 (0,33–0,93)	0,68 (0,34–1,02)	0,75 (0,45–1,05)	0,88 (0,60–1,16)	1,08 (0,70–1,46)
FV (U/mL)	0,72 (0,34–1,08)	0,95 (0,45–1,45)	0,98 (0,62–1,34)	0,90 (0,48–1,32)	0,91 (0,55–1,27)	1,06 (0,62–1,50)
FVII (U/mL)	0,66 (0,28–1,04)	0,89 (0,35–1,43)	0,90 (0,42–1,38)	0,91 (0,39–1,43)	0,87 (0,47–1,27)	1,05 (0,67–1,43)
FVIII (U/mL)	1,00 (0,50–1,78)	0,88 (0,50–1,50)*	0,91 (0,50–1,57)*	0,79 (0,50–1,25)*	0,73 (0,50–109)	0,99 (0,50–1,49)
VWF (U/mL)	1,53 (0,50–2,87)	1,40 (0,50–2,54)	1,28 (0,50–2,46)	1,18 (0,50–2,06)	1,07 (0,50–1,97)	0,92 (0,50–1,58)
FIX (U/mL)	0,53 (0,15–0,91)	0,53 (0,15–0,91)	0,51 (0,21–0,81)	0,67 (0,21–1,13)	0,86 (0,36–1,36)	1,09 (0,55–1,63)
FX (U/mL)	0,40 (0,12–0,68)	0,49 (0,19–0,79)	0,59 (0,31–0,87)	0,71 (0,35–1,07)	0,78 (0,38–1,18)	1,06 (0,70–1,52)
FXI (U/mL)	0,38 (0,10–0,66)	0,55 (0,23–0,87)	0,53 (0,27–0,79)	0,69 (0,41–0,97)	0,86 (0,49–1,34)	0,97 (0,67–1,27)
FXII (U/mL)	0,53 (0,13–0,93)	0,47 (0,11–0,83)	0,49 (0,17–0,81)	0,67 (0,25–1,09)	0,77 (0,39–1,15)	1,08 (0,52–1,64)
Antithrombin (U/mL)	0,63 (0,39–0,87)	0,67 (0,41–0,93)	0,78 (0,48–1,08)	0,97 (0,73–1,21)*	1,04 (0,84–1,24)	1,05 (0,79–1,31)
Protein C (U/mL)	0,35 (0,17–0,53)	0,42 (0,20–0,64)	0,43 (0,21–0,65)	0,54 (0,28–0,80)	0,59 (0,37–0,81)	0,96 (0,64–1,28)

From Am J Pediatr, Hematol, Oncol, 12:95, 1990.

Table 13.2 Some hemostasis variables in healthy children

Variable	1–5 years	6–10 years	11–16 years	Adults
Fibrinogen, g/L	2,76 (1,70–4,00)	2,79 (1,57–4,00)	3,0 (1,54–4,48)	2,78 (1,56–4,00)
Prothrombin, (U/mL)	0,94 (0,71–1,16)*	0,88 (0,67–1,07)*	0,83 (0,61–1,04)*	1,08 (0,70–1,46)
FV, (U/mL)	1,03 (0,79–1,27)	0,90 (0,63–1,16)*	0,77 (0,55–0,99)*	1,06 (0,62–1,50)
FVII, (U/mL)	0,82 (0,55–1,16)*	0,85 (0,52–1,20)*	0,83 (0,58–1,15)*	1,05 (0,67–1,43)
FVIII, (U/mL)	0,90 (0,59–1,42)	0,95 (0,58–1,32)	0,92 (0,53–1,31)	0,99 (0,50–1,49)
VWFag, (U/mL)	0,82 (0,60–1,20)	0,95 (0,44–1,44)	1,00 (0,46–1,53)	0,92 (0,50–1,58)
FIX, (U/mL)	0,73 (0,47–1,04)*	0,75 (0,63–0,89)*	0,82 (0,59–1,22)*	1,09 (0,55–1,63)
FX, (U/mL)	0,88 (0,58–1,16)*	0,75 (0,55–1,01)*	0,79 (0,50–1,17)*	1,06 (0,60–1,52)
FXI, (U/mL)	0,94 (0,56–1,50)	0,86 (0,52–1,20)	0,74 (0,50–0,97)*	0,97 (0,67–1,27)
FXII, (U/mL)	0,93 (0,64–1,29)	0,92 (0,60–1,40)	0,81 (0,34–1,37)*	1,08 (0,52–1,64)
Antithrombin, ag (U/mL)	1,11 (0,82–1,39)	1,11 (0,90–1,31)	1,05 (0,77–1,32)	1,0 (0,74–1,26)
Protein C, ag (U/mL)	0,66 (0,40–0,92)*	0,69 (0,45–0,93)*	0,83 (0,55–1,11)*	0,96 (0,64–1,28)

* The values are significantly different compared to adults

The values, except for fibrinogen are compared with a pooled normal plasma robese 1 mL Contains IU/ML

From Andrew et al., Blood 80 1998, 1992.

concentration of many of the components reaches adult values at the age of 6 months in both premature and full-term children. Newborns have the same number of platelets as adults but platelet function is reduced. In spite of this, newborns have a shorter bleeding time than adults, which can be explained by high levels of VWF (especially the high molecular forms) and high hematocrit. Knowledge of the development of the hemostasis system is of importance for treatment and/or diagnosis in children with bleeding or thrombosis symptoms.

Bleeding in newborns

The most common reasons for bleeding symptoms in newborns are acquired coagulation disturbances caused by asphyxia, infection, liver disease or vitamin K deficiency. For information on disseminated intravascular coagulation (DIC) and liver disease, see Chapter 14.

Vitamin K deficiency bleeding

Hemorrhagic disease of the newborn is caused by reduced transportation of vitamin K through the placenta, small amounts of vitamin K in breast-milk and sterile intestines in newborns. The concentration of the vitamin K-dependent factors (see above) in plasma is low postnatally and these factors are inactive without vitamin K. The bleeding symptoms vary but are often serious, e.g. intracranially or intestinally. The "classic" form starts during the second to third days of life. Early forms beginning during the first 24 hours are rare. They are caused by treatment of the mother with drugs interfering with the vitamin K function, for instance by phenytoin. Late forms starting during weeks 2–8 are caused by dietary factors in combination with malabsorbtion or liver disease. Vitamin K deficiency is rarely seen in children who have had breast milk substitute.

Intramuscular or subcutaneous injection of 1 mg vitamin K prevents the "classic" and late forms of this bleeding tendency. In oral treatment, repeated doses are required in order to prevent development of the late form of vitamin K deficiency bleeding in breastfed children.

Laboratory diagnosis
Elevated PT(INR) (decreased levels of FII, FVII, FIX and FX). More severe forms have a prolonged APT time.

Treatment
Vitamin K (Konakion®); 1 mg intravenously usually normalizes PT(INR) within a few hours. Plasma, about 10 mL/kg, or prothrombin complex concentrates can be necessary for serious bleeding symptoms. Consult coagulation experts about dosage. See Chapter 5.

Hereditary bleeding tendency

In otherwise healthy children with bleeding symptoms, a hereditary bleeding disorder should be suspected. The heredity is essential, but a negative family anamnesis does not exclude a hereditary disorder.

Coagulation factor deficiencies

Hemophilia A and B

The most common forms of hereditary coagulation factor deficiencies are hemophilia A (FVIII deficiency) and hemophilia B (FIX deficiency). Both diseases are inherited sex bound recessively. Today, fetal diagnosis can be offered to almost all possible or known carriers of hemophilia. Hemophilia A is present in about 1/10,000 men and hemophilia B in about 1/30,000 men. Spontaneous mutations are common in hemophilia A.

Diagnosis

Only 15–30% of newborns with hemophilia show bleeding symptoms during the neonatal period. Most are iatrogenic, caused by intramuscular injections (vitamin K), venous sampling (PKU test) or vacuum extraction at birth. Vacuum extraction increases the risk of intracranial bleeding in children with a bleeding disorder and should be avoided at the delivery of children with known hemophilia heredity.

The most common presenting symptom is hematoma, starting when the child becomes more mobile. The hematomas are larger, darker and with a "bumpy" look compared with those in healthy children. The mean age of diagnosis in Sweden is 9 months in the most severe cases of hemophilia. The main symptoms of these forms are joint and muscle bleedings usually appearing at the age of 1–3 years.

Laboratory diagnosis

Activated partial thromboplastin time is prolonged. Note that mild forms of hemophilia can have a normal value for the age. Decreased value of FVIII or FIX verifies the diagnosis. Mild forms of hemophilia B can be difficult to diagnose in newborns, who generally have low levels of FIX. Sampling should be repeated after 6 months of age.

Treatment

In severe hemophilia, preventive treatment (prophylaxis) with factor concentrates should start between 1 and 2 years of age. The children are preferably treated with recombinant factor concentrates. The prophylaxis treatment starts with one injection per week, 250–500 IU. As soon as possible, from a technical and psychologic point of view, the treatment intensity increases to 3–4 times per week in hemophilia A and twice per week in hemophilia B. Pain-relieving treatment with EMLA

(Lidocain-Prilocain) ointment has made it easier to perform intravenous injections and blood sampling by a peripheral vein.

Home treatment, i.e. treatment performed by the parents, is usually started after 16–18 months of treatment in the pediatric outpatient clinic. Children showing repeated bleeding symptoms and those in whom peripheral vein injections have not been successful are given an implantable venous access system (Port-A-Cath). Early onset of prophylaxis treatment has meant that most children grow up without permanent joint damage. Quality of life has been improved with less (or no) absence from school and the possibility of joining in physical activities with children of the same age.

Operations in children with most bleeding disorders can be performed today for the same indications as in healthy children. However, they should be performed in hospitals with coagulation expertise.

The most serious complication of treatment with factor concentrate is the development of antibodies against the coagulation factor in question. Antibodies against FVIII occur in 10–30% of children with hemophilia A, most commonly in those with severe forms. They often appear early (after less than 50 injections). Antibodies against FIX are more rare but in contrast to the FVIII inhibitors, administration of FIX concentrate to these patients can result in serious allergic side effects, even anaphylaxis.

High levels of antibodies FVIII or FIX make it impossible to treat bleeding or give bleeding prophylaxis with FVIII or FIX concentrates For elimination of antibodies (tolerance induction) and treatment of bleedings, see Chapter 4.

Tranexamic acid (Cyklokapron®) is used for minor bleeding symptoms, especially in mucous membranes. The youngest children are given a mixture 100 mg/mL (extempore preparation). Recommended oral dose is 20 mg/kg bodyweight three times daily. For IV treatment we recommend 10 mg/kg bodyweight three times in 24 hours.

VWD

Severe forms of this disease can cause bleeding problems during the neonatal period. The most common, i.e. mild, forms are difficult to diagnose at this age, as high levels of FVIII and VWF are physiologic during the neonatal period. These patients are usually diagnosed later in life or before starting school due to epistaxis and/or hematomas.

Blood sampling is appropriate after 3 months of age in children with bleeding symptoms or known heredity.

Laboratory diagnosis
See Chapters 3 and 4.

Treatment
See Chapter 4.

Rare hereditary forms

These are usually autosomally recessively inherited. In severe deficiency of fibrinogen, FVII, FX and FXIII, bleeding symptoms are frequent in the neonatal stage. Bleeding from the umbilical cord is seen in 80% of children with severe FXIII deficiency and is also common in severe FX deficiency. In these deficiencies there is a great risk of intracranial bleedings during childhood. FXIII deficiency also leads to muscular bleeding symptoms, impaired wound-healing capacity and increased frequency of repeated spontaneous abortions.

Laboratory diagnosis

For evaluation of APT time and PT(INR) see Chapter 3. Note that FXIII deficiency does not affect APT time or PT(INR). The diagnoses are established by analyses of the respective factors.

Treatment

Substitution with plasma (10–15 mL/kg bodyweight) or if available with factor concentrate (e.g. fibrinogen, FXIII, FVII). The treatment is given at bleeding or as prophylaxis, depending on the frequency and characteristics of the bleeding.

Platelet function defect

The symptoms are similar to those in VWD and should be suspected in children with mucocutaneous bleedings or with a tendency to hematomas. Such defects are often hereditary. More severe forms are rare (e.g. Glanzmann's thrombasthenia and Bernard–Soulier syndrome) and symptoms can occur during the first year of life.

Diagnosis and treatment

See Chapter 4.

Acquired bleeding tendency

Thrombocytopenia

The number of platelets in healthy newborns is comparable with adults. Thrombocytopenia is often seen in severely ill newborns. Most frequent symptoms are bleedings from skin and mucous membranes. Tranexamic acid (Cyklokapron®) usually has a good effect on these symptoms. Platelet infusion is needed at low levels (below $20 \times 10^9/L$) and serious bleedings or in combination with other bleeding disposing factors.

Acute idiopathic thrombocytopenic purpura

Idiopathic thrombocytopenic purpura is caused by autoimmune antibodies against the glycoproteins of the platelet membranes. The disease can start after a viral infection. Mild bleeding symptoms can be treated as detailed above. Intracranial bleedings rarely occur.

These patients are usually investigated by hematologists. Treatment consists of steroids (1–2 mg/kg bodyweight) or γ-globulin IV (0.4 g/kg bodyweight for 5 days). Platelet transfusions should only be given in cases with severe bleeding symptoms. The prognosis is usually good.

Hemolytic uremic syndrome and thrombotic thrombocytopenic purpura
See Chapter 14.

Bleeding tendency secondary to liver or kidney diseas
See Chapter 5.

Thromboembolic disorders in children

Thrombotic diseases in children are different from those of adults in many ways. The incidence is significantly lower and thrombosis prophylaxis is therefore not considered adequate for children in connection with, for example, orthopedic surgery. Children with hereditary prothrombotic risk factors do not usually develop thrombosis until in the upper teens or as adults. The low incidence has resulted in a low number of patients in the studies performed on diagnosis and treatment of thromboembolism in children. The incidence of symptom-producing venous thrombosis is reported to be 0.07/10,000 children and for hospitalized children about 5.3/10,000. Newborns have the greatest risk of thromboembolic complications.

Recommendations concerning diagnosis and treatment have to a great extent been based on experience in adults. Acquired risk factors, such as malignancy, infection, heart disease or indwelling catheters, are common in children developing thrombosis. Newborns have about 50% of adult levels of the three prothrombotic risk factors (inhibitors) – antithrombin (AT), protein C and protein S – the latter two being vitamin K dependent, which makes it difficult to diagnose familiar deficiencies in children before 6 months of age. Also the presence of FV Leiden mutation or prothrombin mutation might increase the risks.

The treatment of thrombosis is also affected by lower thrombin generation in children and by low levels of plasminogen in newborns. Several studies have shown an increased presence of cardiolipin/lupus antibodies in children with a thrombotic disease and idiopathic cerebral ischemia. There is an ongoing discussion on whether or not this is a risk factor for thrombosis in children or an epiphenomenon.

Venous thrombosis

An underlying disease is usually present in children who develop thrombosis. Idiopathic venous thrombosis occurs in less than 5% of the children compared with about 40% in adults. The majority of the children have several risk factors, the most important of which is an indwelling catheter (observed in 90% of children with venous thrombosis during the neonatal period and in 66% of patients with venous thrombosis during childhood). This fact also explains why thrombosis in the upper venous system is so common in children (60%) compared with adults (2%). There are no differences in incidence between the sexes.

Kidney vein thrombosis is the most common type of noncatheter-related venous thrombosis in the youngest children. Symptoms in newborns are palpable resistance in the flank, hematuria, proteinuria and thrombocytopenia. Children under 1 year of age usually present with symptoms such as diarrhea, vomiting and dehydration.

The incidence of pulmonary embolism in children is not known but possibly underestimated. These children most often have multiple risk factors for thrombosis, of which the most important is a central venous line.

The risk of recurrence in children is reported to be about 8%, and 10–20% of the children develop post-thrombotic symptoms. The mortality directly related to thrombosis or pulmonary embolism is suggested to be 20%.

Diagnosis
For physical and radiologic investigations, see Chapter 7.

Treatment
The choice of treatment drugs and treatment time is based on studies in adults with a thrombotic disease. UFH and LMH are used to about the same extent. There has been a gradual increase in the use of LMH due to more predictable pharmacokinetics, reduced requirement for monitoring and possibly fewer complications.

UFH
Evaluation of the effect in newborns is difficult because of their immature hemostatic system and low levels of antithrombin, possibly resulting in less effect. Half-life for UFH in blood is 1–2 hours in older children, but has been reported to be as low as 25 minutes in the newborn.
- Recommended dose: bolus 75 U/kg bodyweight.
- Maintainance dose: children younger than 1 year – 28 U/kg bodyweight. For children older than 1 year – 20 U/kg bodyweight an hour. Aim for an APT time 2–3 times prolongation of the upper limit of APT time.

LMH
Dose studies in children have been performed primarily with enoxaparin (Klexane®). Dalteparin (Fragmin®) has also been used. The drug is given subcutaneously. It is excreted through the kidneys and can consequently accumulate in kidney failure (clearance below 30 mL/min). LMH does not affect the APT time to the same degree as UHF. The effect of LMH is preferably monitored by determination of anti-FXa about 3–4 hours after the third-fourth injection. The aim is a level of 0.5–1.0 anti-FXa. Half-life for LMH SC is 3–4 hours.

Recommended dose (treatment)
- *Klexane*. Age below 2 months, 1.5 mg/kg bodyweight sc twice daily. Age more than 2 months, 1.0 mg/kg bodyweight sc twice daily.
- *Fragmin*. Age below 2 months, 125 U/kg bodyweight sc twice daily. Age more than 2 months, 100 U/kg bodyweight sc twice daily.

When the situation is stable, the drugs can be given once/24 hours.
- *Klexane:* 1.5 mg/kg bodyweight sc once/24 hours.
- *Fragmin:* 200 U/kg bodyweight sc once/24 hours.

If continued treatment with LMH is planned without change to warfarin or other AVK drug, the dose can be changed after a few weeks to:
- *Klexane:* 1 mg/kg bodyweight sc once/24 hours
- *Fragmin:* 125 U/kg bodyweight sc once/24 hours.

Prophylaxis against venous thrombosis is rarely given to children. The documentation is not sufficient.

Bleeding complications during treatment with UFH and LMH
and warfarin
Protamine neutralizes the anticoagulation effect of UFH and to some degree the effect of LMH. 1 mg protamine neutralizes 100–150 units of UFH. The effect is temporary and can be monitored with APT time when using UFH. It should only be used in patients with serious bleeding symptoms. See Chapter 5.

Heparin-induced thrombocytopenia
The incidence heparin-induced thrombocytopenia in UFH-treated children is not known. For diagnosis and treatment of HIT, see Chapter 14.

Treatment with AVK drugs
The effect of these drugs is mediated by competitive blocking of the vitamin K metabolism. This leads to decreasing plasma levels of FII, FVII, FIX and FX and consequently an elevated PT(INR) within 1–3 days of

beginning treatment. The treatment is usually given orally once a day, but can be given IV.

Newborns have physiologically low levels and are seldom treated with AVK drugs.

Dosage

Day 1: 0.2 mg/kg bodyweight, maintaining this dose day 2–3 or until PT(INR) is >1.4. Thereafter 50% of the initial dose until PT(INR) is in the therapeutic interval usually 2–3. The dose is therefore reduced usually reduced to 25% of the initial dose.

If PT(INR) is over 3.5, the dose is reduced after 1–2 days' interruption of treatment with the drug. Older children and teenagers often need a lower dose (0.1 mg/kg bodyweight).

Prothrombin complex concentrates and plasma can be used to reduce PT(INR) if needed because of bleeding symptom or the necessity of acute surgery

Aim

Level of PT(INR) during continuous treatment is 2–3; at high risk of bleeding, 2.0.

To reverse a high PT(INR) see Chapter 8. Note that PT(INR) reversal is faster in newborns.

Duration of anticoagulation treatment

The recommended treatment of newborns is usually UFH or LMH for 10–14 days. For older children, treatment with an AVK drug or LMH for 3–6 months is recommended after the first thrombosis or pulmonary embolism.

Long-term treatment, usually with an AVK drug and with a yearly evaluation of continuing therapy, might be necessary for children with recurrence or serious thrombotic disease, including remaining risk factors. In children, monitoring of PT(INR) is recommended at least every fourth week.

Sinusvenous thrombosis

The etiology of sinusvenous thrombosis in children is unclear, and the importance of prothrombotic risk factors generating the disease is not known. Half the number of children with a sinus thrombosis develop secondary cerebral infarction as a result of rapid thrombotic development and a total venous occlusion. Fifty percent of these cases are found in newborns and preschool children. The symptoms are often discrete and develop over several days (headache, nausea, apathia). Seizures are common in the youngest children. Newborns show a tense fontanelle and possibly enlarged scalp veins and swollen eyelids.

The majority of children (65%) have at least two risk factors, such as otitis media, sinuitis, trauma, dehydration or heart failure. Rheumatoid arthritis, SLE and chronic intestinal disease are more common in older children. Acquired and hereditary prothrombotic risk factors may possibly contribute to the origin of sinus thrombosis. The most common of these risk factors is the presence of cardiolipin/lupus antibodies. Mortality is still about 10%. 50–75% of children recover. The remaining patients have neurologic sequelae.

Diagnosis
Best performed by magnetic resonance imaging. See Chapter 7.

Treatment
Most of the children receive anticoagulation treatment with UFH/LMH followed by an AVK drug for 3–6 months. The recommendations are based on studies in adult patients. Newborns without large cerebral bleeding symptoms can be treated with UFH or LMH for 10–14 days. Local thrombolytic treatment has been used in a few patients with progressive symptoms in spite of anticoagulation treatment.

Thrombolytic treatment
Thrombolytic drugs act by transforming endogenous plasminogen to plasmin. Since newborns have a reduced level of plasminogen (about 50% that of adults) such drugs might be less effective. Currently we recommend alteplase (Actilyse®) for thrombolytic treatment in connection with massive pulmonary embolism or extended thrombosis in children who do not respond to treatment with UFH or LMH. In minor studies, Actilyse 0.1–0.5 mg/kg/h for 6 hours has been used. Lower doses for a longer treatment period up to 3 days has also been effective. Usually the treatment is combined with UFH and plasma. Always consult coagulation experts. The thrombolytic effect can be followed by measuring fibrinogen and fibrin D-dimer. The same contraindications apply as in adults (see Chapter 8). Bleeding complications are common in children (68%). Bleeding necessitating transfusion occurs in 39%. For treatment of bleeding in connection with thrombolysis, see Chapter 8.

Investigation of prothrombotic risk factors
An investigation usually can be performed 3–6 months after the thrombosis event. A venous thrombosis in children, producing symptoms, most often has a multifactorial genesis. Hereditary or acquired deficiencies of coagulation inhibitors AT, protein C, protein S (free fraction), presence of FV mutation (1691G>A), prothrombin polymorphism (20210G>A), increased levels of homocysteine and lipoprotein (a) or

acquired phospholipid antibodies have all been associated with increased risk of venous thrombosis.

Arterial thrombosis

Arterial thrombosis is rare in otherwise healthy children. It usually occurs in connection with arterial catheterizing in heart disorders and in newborns with a umbilical arterial catheter.

Recommendations concerning diagnosis and treatment of these thromboses are based on studies in adults. A preventive treatment is often given with UFH in connection with heart catheterization. A bolus dose with 100–150 U/kg bodyweight reduced thromboembolic complications from 40% to 8%. Long-term treatment with an AVK drug such as warfarin or ASA is usually given to children with complicated heart disease or after heart surgery.

The incidence of thromboembolism in connection with a umbillical arterial catheter varies depending on examination techniques (10–60%). The symptoms depend on the extension of the thrombosis. Many newborns are asymptomatic, while others show a serious ischemia in legs and other organs (1–5%). Prophylactic treatment with low doses of UFH (1–5 U/h) is often given to newborns with an arterial catheter. In addition to removal of the catheter, treatment with UFH is recommended. In connection with aorta thrombosis, thrombolysis with t-PA (Actilyse) may be required.

Children with Kawasaki's disease are initially treated with high doses of ASA (80–100 mg/kg bodyweight/day) during the first weeks, and thereafter a lower dose (3–5 mg/kg bodyweight/day) during the following 7 weeks or longer.

Stroke

Stroke in children is rare compared with adults. The incidence is stated to be about 8 per 100,000 children/year. The ratio of arterial ischemic stroke to sinus thrombosis is 3:1. A third of the children with stroke are affected during the neonatal period. The incidence of stroke during childhood seems to increase, probably due to improved imaging diagnosis and increased survival of children with severe heart diseases, malignancies and pronounced prematurity.

Ischemic stroke

Ischemic stroke in children is usually caused by an embolus or a local thrombosis formation. In 25% of cases, the source of embolism is the heart, e.g. atrial septal defect or open foramen ovale with a right-to-left shunt or cardiac surgery. Most cases with ischemic stroke are found in newborns and small children. The most common symptom to start with is seizures. Small children suffer from headache, sickness and fever. In older children, seizures and hemiparesis are the most common symptoms.

Risk factors
Heart disease, sickle cell anemia, trauma of head or neck causing dissection of the vessel wall, vasculitis (varicella infection, radiation therapy, Takayasu's arteritis, Moyamoya's syndrome) hereditary or acquired prothrombotic risk factors. The latter (see above) is found in about 30%.

Diagnosis
Computed tomography, magnetic resonance imaging and angiography.

Treatment
The risk/benefit ratio of antithrombotic treatment of stroke in children is not known. There are currently no controlled studies. About 35–65% of children with arterial ischemic stroke are treated with UFH, LMH, AVK drug (warfarin) or ASA. Thrombolytic treatment is rare. Children are rarely diagnosed within 3 hours of the first symptom, which is recommended in adults for this type of treatment.

The risk of bleeding complications in children receiving thrombolytic treatment has not been evaluated. In newborns who have-the highest incidence of stroke, less effect can be expected due to low levels of plasminogen.

Anticoagulant treatment with UFH/LMH for 3 months is recommended in newborns with a source of cardiac emboli. Usually no treatment is given to other cases. For older children we recommend UFH/LMH for 5–7 days or until the cause of the stroke has been established. Thereafter ASA (2–5 mg/kg/bodyweight/day) is recommended, based on studies in adults. New types of platelet inhibitors, such as clopidogrel, have not been studied in children. In children with cardiac embolic sources, warfarin is often used for long-term prophylaxis.

Prognosis
Retrospective studies show neurologic sequelae in three-quarters of the children. In one study 37% of the children were shown to totally recover, 46% showed mild to moderate neurologic sequelae and 16% had more severe sequelae. The risk of recurrence is stated to be 15–20% (most occurs in children with heart diseases).

Emergency conditions associated with coagulation activation

CHAPTER 14

Jovan P. Antovic[1] and Margareta Holmström[2]

[1]Department of Molecular Medicine and Surgery, Coagulation Research, Karolinska Institutet, Stockholm, Sweden, [2]Department of Medicine, Coagulation Unit, Karolinska Institutet, Hematology Centre, Karolinska University Hospital Solna, Stockholm, Sweden

Disseminated intravascular coagulation

Definition

Disseminated intravascular coagulation (DIC) was defined by the DIC Subcommittee of the Scientific and Standardization Committee of the International Society of Hemostasis and Thrombosis in 2001 as follows: "DIC is an acquired syndrome characterized by the intravascular activation of coagulation with loss of localization arising from different causes. It can originate from and cause damage to the microvasculature, which, if sufficiently severe, can produce organ dysfunction."

Pathophysiology

Disseminated intravascular coagulation is induced by numerous factors in which tissue damage, endothelial damage or damage to blood cells have a central role. Examples of cell-damaging mediators are endo- and exotoxins from bacteria, antigen-antibody complexes, cytokines released from macrophages and monocytes, proteases released from white blood cells, etc.

Tissue factor is exposed on and/or released from damaged tissue, endothelial cells or monocytes. The amount of released tissue factor is related to subsequent coagulation activation. DIC is characterized by a primary hypercoagulation phase with disseminated intravascular fibrin formation and microembolism.

Essential Guide to Blood Coagulation. By Jovan P. Antovic and Margareta Blombäck
© Blackwell Publishing, ISBN: 9781405196277

Soluble fibrin complexes in the circulation precipitate and form, together with platelets (and leukocytes), thromboemboli in the microcirculation, resulting in organ damage. All organ systems can be affected: kidneys, lungs and the central nervous system are particularly sensitive. Microembolism is considered to be one component of the syndrome, usually characterized by a progressive development of multiple organ failure (MOF). The hypercoagulation results in consumption of coagulation factors, inhibitors and platelets. Consumption is faster than synthesis.

Secondarily, there is also a physiologic activation of other proteolytic enzyme systems, including formation of elastase and plasmin, leading to an increased fibrinolysis, with degradation of fibrinogen, fibrin, other coagulation factors and receptors on the platelet surface. The stimulation of fibrinolysis results in raised concentrations of fibrin(ogen) degradation products (FDP), including fibrin D-dimers, that inhibit fibrin formation and platelet aggregation. A paradoxic combination of microembolism and bleeding (thrombohemorrhagic syndrome) may occur.

Secondary activation of, for example, complement and kallikrein-kinin systems is of great pathophysiologic importance and possibly also for therapy.

In certain cases, inhibition of fibrinolysis occurs simultaneously with activation of the coagulation system. There are specific diseases in which fibrinolysis may dominate, e.g. promyelocytic leukemia.

Examples of conditions triggering DIC

Sepsis, trauma (including burns and heat stroke), particularly head and polytrauma, obstetric complications, malignancy, toxins (e.g. snake venom), immunologic/allergic disorders, vascular disorders (e.g. aneurysm).

The clinical picture

Typical symptoms of DIC emanate from the most sensitive organs, i.e. the central nervous system, kidneys, lungs, skin and mucous membranes. Symptoms may be trivial at an early stage, but fulminant multiorgan failure may occur in later stages, including significant cerebral symptoms, acute lung failure (acute respiratory distress syndrome), renal failure, and also necrosis of skin and mucous membranes due to the microthrombosis. Coagulation activation associated with microthrombosis may be unrecognized in the early stages and/or misdiagnosed as complications of underlying disease, and suspicion of DIC may be established only when bleedings occur. Petechial bleedings and ecchymoses as well as mucosal bleeding from gums etc. and bleedings from venous punctures and catheter sites are the most common findings. Gastrointestinal bleeding may occur as well as intracranial bleedings.

In **septic shock**, a severe form of DIC, powerful activation of the coagulation often occurs very quickly, mainly through upregulation of tissue factor from damaged endothelium and monocytes. Fibrinolysis is inhibited. In meningococcal sepsis, for example, blue-black confluent skin changes are found, due to a combination of necrosis and bleeding.

Laboratory diagnosis of DIC

Disseminated intravascular coagulation develops in stages and the diagnosis (and treatment) differs accordingly.

1. Generalized activation of coagulation, with intravascular formation of soluble fibrin.
2. Consumption of platelets, coagulation factors and inhibitors. Secondary fibrinolysis.
3. Microembolism and/or bleeding in various organs.
4. Multiple organ failure may develop as a result of uninhibited DIC.

Laboratory values change. Repeat the analyses to identify trends.

- *Platelet count* decreases due to consumption.
- *APT time* is prolonged after consumption. Pathologic test results occur relatively late in the process, when general factor deficiency such as of FVIII and/or fibrinogen has reached about 30% of normal values.
- *Low EVF* (Hct <20%) leads to prolonged P-APT time.
- *PT(INR)* increases as the vitamin K-dependent coagulation factors are consumed. Liver failure may interfere with the evaluation of laboratory data. Pathologic test results occur relatively late in the process, when general factor deficiency has reached about 30% of normal values.
- *Fibrinogen* may drop, due to rapid fibrin formation and degradation, but its level can also be normal or high, especially in an infection, since fibrinogen is an acute phase reactant. At a level below 1 g/L bleeding often starts. Therefore repetitive measurements of fibrinogen should be performed. Fibrinogen <0.5 g/L results in a prolonged APT time.
- *Fibrin D-dimer* usually increases, indicating fibrin formation followed by subsequent fibrinolysis.
- *Antithrombin* is consumed as a result of increased thrombin formation. It also can drop due to being dependent on liver function.
- *Soluble fibrin*, an intermediate stage between fibrinogen and stable (crossbound) fibrin, increases when the formation of fibrin is stimulated.

Treatment monitoring

Use laboratory tests to evaluate progress and treatment. Repeat testing 2–4 times daily.

Platelet count, APT time, PT(INR), fibrinogen, fibrin D-dimer, antithrombin 2–3 times per day.

If bleeding symtoms are, fibrinogen and FVIII concentrations need to be analyzed. Special tests may be suggested by coagulation specialists.

Treatment

It is mandatory to treat the underlying cause of DIC, e.g. treatment of infection, fracture stabilization, emptying of abscesses, debridement of necrotic tissue, delivery induction or caesarean section in obstetric complications, etc. Without treatment and cure of the cause, DIC will not subside.

As this treatment policy is now more widely applied, DIC does not occur so often.

General treatment for sepsis

General recommendations focus on rapid diagnosis and treatment of the cause, i.e. give adequate antibiotics in combination with shock therapy and support of vital functions. No tranexamic acid as fibrinolysis usually is impaired.

Specific treatment of coagulation disturbances

The specific treatment of DIC is mainly based on clinical experience and physiologic considerations arising from studies in animals. However, the positive effects of various treatment options in animal studies have not been confirmed in human studies, probably because patients with DIC are so heterogeneous and the causes of DIC multifactorial.

Substitution of acquired deficiencies of inhibitors of coagulation, fibrinolysis and kallikrein is usually initially achieved with plasma transfusion. If volume needs to be limited, plasma may be replaced by inhibitor and/or factor concentrates. Platelet count may be transfused if platelet count is very low ($<20 \times 10^9/L$) in combination with persistent bleeding. Discuss with coagulation specialist. For details see below.

When DIC subsides, antithrombotic treatment (LMH) may be considered.

Caution
- LMH creates an increased bleeding tendency, which should be considered in particular if platelet count is low (below $20 \times 10^9/L$) and there is ongoing bleeding.
- Patients with traumatic brain injury may be given LMH in prophylactic doses 24 hours after injury if there is no obvious ongoing bleeding or contraindication. Brain injury is a potent activator of coagulation.
- LMH can cause thrombocytopenia due to antibodies against platelet factor 4. See below.

- Accumulation of heparins may occur in renal and hepatic insufficiency. Consider dose reduction if increased creatinine or pathologic liver tests.
- The plasma activity of heparin can be monitored by measuring anti-FXa.

Fresh-stored (less than 2 weeks) or fresh-frozen plasma
This is first option *in* bleeding. The plasma is given to supply coagulation, fibrinolysis and other protease inhibitors. In the absence of dilution, a general inhibitory deficiency may be presumed if antithrombin levels are low. Fifteen mL plasma/kg bodyweight will increase the levels of inhibitors and coagulation factors by about 10–15%.

Antithrombin concentrate
The half-life of antithrombin is normally 3 days, but in DIC it can be 4–24 hours.

A large randomized study (Kybersept), did not show any significant effects on **septic patients** of treatment with antithrombin concentrate. However, there is a relatively long clinical experience with antithrombin treatment in patients with septic shock and severe progressive coagulopathy despite large plasma supply. Appropriate patients for this type of treatment may be those with fulminant septic shock caused by meningococci or pneumococci and symptoms of coagulopathy in the form of purpura or other bleedings.

Only a low antithrombin level is not an indication for antithrombin treatment. Heparin should be avoided together with antithrombin infusion due to the increased risk of bleeding.

Note that the combination of LMH and substitution of antithrombin may lead to an amplified anticoagulation effect and increased bleeding.

Coagulation factor concentrates
These can be used in severe DIC with consumption of the factors, especially FVIII, fibrinogen and FXIII. Factor concentrates should preferably not be substituted until the pathologic consumptive hypercoagulation ("fuel on the fire") has ceased and there is still bleeding due to low levels of factors. Patients needing factor concentrate often have a spontaneously prolonged APT time.

- *Vitamin-K dependent factor concentrates.* Nonactivated prothrombin complex concentrates of factors II, VII, IX, X, protein C and protein S are used in serious bleedings as well as when PT(INR) exceeds 1.6 (preferred level in surgical hemostasis) or plasma treatment is not sufficient. The effect is instantaneous and lasts for 6–12 hours.

- *Fibrinogen concentrate* is used in serious bleedings, at fibrinogen concentrations <1 g/L and when plasma administration is not sufficient or difficult to perform. One gram of the concentrate increases the fibrinogen level by 0.3 g/L in an adult. For full hemostasis effect a level of 2 g/L or more is needed if the patient is bleeding. Half-life (normally 4.5 days) is shorter in massive hypercoagulation including consumption and degradation.
- VWF/factor VIII concentrate (Haemate®). In conditions involving massive fibrinolysis, it is not just fibrinogen that is degraded but also FVIII, VWF and FXIII. A low FVIII level causes a prolonged APT time and low VWF causes a prolonged bleeding time and worsened primary hemostasis. Haemate may be indicated in massive fibrinolysis and/or serious bleeding problems which are not improved by plasma (and eventually platelet concentrate).

Recombinant human activated protein C (rhAPC) (Xigris®)

Recombinant human activated protein C has been shown *experimentally* to inhibit coagulation and inflammation and can stimulate fibrinolysis. The immune-modulating effect is probably of greater importance than the effect on coagulation. In a large, randomized clinical study (PROWESS) in severe sepsis, a 6.1% mortality reduction was found after 28 days with rhAPC treatment compared to placebo.

In serious bleeding or prior to invasive surgery, the treatment should be interrupted and the effect of rhAPC will rapidly diminish. Contraindications and warnings must be carefully considered, as the treatment is associated with an increased risk of serious bleeding. Take special care in patients with low fibrinogen level and platelet count and/or high PT(INR). There are, however, many contraindications for rhAPC treatment that exclude septic patients and there is still substantial skepticism surrounding its efficacy and safety.

Dextran, ASA and NSAID

These may potentiate the risk of bleeding by inhibiting platelet function.

Tranexamic acid (Cyklokapron®)

If, in spite of plasma supply, severe bleeding continues with a low fibrinogen level and continuously high fibrin D-dimer levels, this indicates fibrinolysis. Tranexamic acid 10–15 mg/kg bodyweight IV during protective LMH treatment may be an option, possibly in repeated doses. Be restrictive in the event of a simultaneous massive coagulation activation and in thrombosis. There is a risk that lysis of the microthromboses will cease, followed by remaining organ damage.

In **septic coagulopathy**, treatment with fibrinolysis inhibitors, e.g. tranexamic acid, should be avoided because fibrinolysis is often already inhibited.

Local treatment
Biologic tissue glue, Tisseel®, contains mainly fibrinogen, fibronectin, FXIII, aprotinin and thrombin. Tranexamic acid locally may be effective. The IV preparation is diluted 1 + 1 with physiologic NaCl solution.

Heparin-induced thrombocytopenia

HIT type 1
Heparin-induced thrombocytopenia 1 is a nonimmunologically conditional, benign form of thrombocytopenia occurring during treatment with UFH/LMH. It does not require treatment. It needs to be differentiated from "false thrombocytopenia" which can be diagnosed by measuring platelet count in a test tube with EDTA and comparing it with a tube containing citrate.

HIT type 2
Heparin-induced thrombocytopenia type 2 (usually named HIT only) is a severe, potentially limb- and life-threatening immune-mediated adverse

Table 14.1 Proposed dosages in the treatment of coagulation disturbances in DIC

Drug	Dose
Plasma (not necessarily frozen)	15 mL/kg (elevated PT(INR) drops fresh about 50%) (kg bodyweight × (1.0 U/mL – actual AT level) × 100 , IV
Prothrombin complex concentrate	10 U/kg IV (PT(INR) drops about 50%)
Tranexamic acid (Cyklokapron)	10 mg/kg IV may be repeated × 3. Stop when the bleeding has ceased. Be cautious in kidney damage. Dose adjustment
Other factor concentrates	Contact coagulation expert
Platelet concentrate	Contact coagulation expert
Dalteparin (Fragmin)	2500–5000 IU/d SC
Enoxaparin (Klexane)	20–40 mg/d SC

drug reaction to UFH and/or LMH which occurs in up to 3% of treated patients. In spite of thrombocytopenia, which occurs typically 5–10 days after the initiation of heparin treatment, bleeding is uncommon, while thromboembolic complications are the main clinical problem in patients with HIT.

Heparin-induced thrombocytopenia is caused by the formation of antibodies that activate platelets following heparin administration, with a complex of heparin and platelet factor 4 (PF4) as a principal antigen. The complex links to the FcγRII receptor on the surface of the platelet. In this way, platelet activation and aggregation are induced, leading to thrombosis.

Heparin-induced thrombocytopenia is a clinicopathologic syndrome and diagnosis of HIT primarily remains clinical, supported by confirmatory laboratory testing. The pretest clinical probability scoring system (4Ts) seems to be a valuable tool for HIT diagnosis (Table 14.2).

Table 14.2 The pretest clinical probability (4Ts) score

	Points (0, 1 or 2 for each category: maximum possible score = 8)		
	2	**1**	**0**
Thrombocytopenia	50% fall or platelet nadir 20–100 × 10⁹/L	30–50% fall or platelet nadir 10–20 × 10⁹/L	Fall <30% or platelet nadir <10 × 10⁹/L
Timing of platelet count fall or other sequelae	Clear onset between day 5-day 10; or less than 1 day (if heparin exposure within past 100 days)	Consistent with immunization but not clear (e.g. missing platelet counts) or onset of thrombocytopenia after day 10	Platelet count fall too early (without recent heparin exposure)
Thrombosis or other sequelae (e.g. skin lesions)	New thrombosis; skin necrosis; post heparin bolus acute systemic reaction	Progressive or recurrent thrombosis; erythematous skin lesions; suspected thrombosis not yet proven	None
Other cause for thrombocytopenia not evident	No other cause for platelet count fall is evident	Possible other cause is evident	Definite other cause is present

Pretest clinical probability score: 6–8 = high; 4–5 = intermediate; 0–3 = low.
Lo GK et al. J Thromb Haemost 2006; 4: 759–65.

Diagnosis

A significant decrease in platelet count is a clinical criterion of suspected HIT type 2. It usually occurs when treatment with UFH/LMH has been in progress for 5–14 days. If the patient has been treated with UFH/LMH during the previous 3 months, thrombocytopenia may occur immediately at the start of therapy. In very rare cases, HIT type 2 appears long after the end of treatment with UFH. Platelet count usually returns to normal when treatment with UFH/LMH has ceased. Thrombotic complications may occur.

Other reasons for thrombocytopenia should be excluded.

Laboratory diagnosis of HIT relies on the detection of antibodies against heparin/PF4 complex in plasma or serum with functional and/or immunologic methods. See Chapter 3.

Treatment

Patients being treated with UFH/LMH need anticoagulation in spite of suspected HIT type 2 as they have a paradoxically increased risk of both venous and arterial thrombosis despite decreased platelet count. AVK drugs should not immediately be substituted for UFH/LMH because there is a risk of skin necrosis and should not be given before platelet count is stable at over 100×10^9/L.

Argatroban has been used for a long time in the US for HIT type 2. Danaparoid (currently not available in Sweden) can be used but there is a small risk of cross-reactivity with UFH/LMH with rise of antibody formation and platelet aggregation. The clearance rates of danaparoid and fondaparinux are dependent of renal function, while the clearance of argatroban is dependent on the patient's liver function.

If HIT type 2 is suspected, consult coagulation experts concerning alternative treatment.

Thrombotic microangiopathies (TTP and HUS)

TTP and HUS

In both TTP and HUS, platelets are consumed as platelet aggregates are formed by the interaction of platelets with VWF. The most likely reason is endothelial damage, but the pathogenesis is not totally clear. A big multimer variant of VWF, normally degraded by a metalloprotease (ADAMTS13), has been observed in plasma in TTP. The cause of TTP is infection or autoimmunity (isolated cases); for HUS, it is most often infection (especially shigatoxin-producing *E. coli* in children).

Acquired TTP and HUS are idiopathic in about 80%, and in 20% of TTP secondary to another condition, e.g. infection, cancer, cytostatic and immunosuppressive treatment, bone marrow transplantation and pregnancy. Congenital TTP with deficiency of ADAMTS13 may occur (recurrent cases).

The clinical picture includes thrombocytopenia, hemolytic anemia (elevated LD, increased numbers of reticulocytes, elevated bilirubin and reduced haptoglobin), fragmented erythrocytes in peripheral blood (so-called schistocytes), kidney failure (worse in HUS), fever (mostly in TTP) and neurologic symptoms (particularly in TTP). Diarrhea is frequent when the cause is infection. Coagulation factors are usually not affected, in contrast to DIC. Determination of the ADAMTS13 concentration is not routine and is done only in special laboratories.

Treatment is based on fresh-frozen plasma and plasmapheresis (in hereditary deficiency there are additional possibilities). In autoimmune TTP, chemotherapy may be necessary to prevent recurrence. Without treatment, the prognosis is very serious; with plasmapheresis, however, 80% remission has been reported in idiopathic TTP.

Contact a hematologist, coagulation expert or blood center for advice.

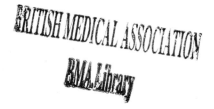

Index

Page numbers in **bold** represent tables, those in *italics* represent figures.